Dependent Agency in the Global
Health Regime

Emma-Louise Anderson • Amy S. Patterson

Dependent Agency in the Global Health Regime

Local African Responses to Donor AIDS Efforts

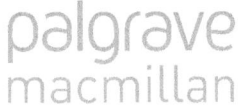

palgrave
macmillan

Emma-Louise Anderson
University of Leeds
Leeds, United Kingdom

Amy S. Patterson
University of the South
Sewanee, Tennessee, USA

ISBN 978-1-137-58147-1   ISBN 978-1-137-58148-8 (eBook)
DOI 10.1057/978-1-137-58148-8

Library of Congress Control Number: 2016952419

Cover illustration: Pattern adapted from an Indian cotton print produced in the 19th century

Printed on acid-free paper

This Palgrave Macmillan imprint is published by Springer Nature
The registered company is Nature America Inc.
The registered company address is: 1 New York Plaza, New York, NY 10004, U.S.A.

To Isabel, Sophia, Neil, Max, and Alex,
With love and gratitude

ACKNOWLEDGMENTS

This project had its roots in pure luck. Both of us attended the 2014 International Studies Association (ISA) conference, each presenting a paper on community responses to donor AIDS programs in Africa. Not knowing one another before the conference, we just happened to read each other's conference papers. As we did, we noticed many similarities: our respondents talked about AIDS donor programs using the same jargon; they exhibited both dependence on global aid structures and an uncanny ability to maneuver around those structures; they challenged how we as political scientists thought about the structure–agency debate. The more we discussed our fieldwork, the more we knew we wanted to write a book that analyzed the "back story" of donor AIDS programs. That is, we wanted to see the ways that local people—often described as "victims," "helpless," and "dependent"—demonstrated autonomy in their actions and reactions as they were caught up in the highly funded donor AIDS programs in Malawi and Zambia. As we each recounted stories of these dependent agents, we began to ask: What makes such agency possible? And why might it matter? Over the course of working together we have been fortunate that we have been able to "pick up the slack" for one another when other projects, family obligations, and teaching requirements drew our attention from the book.

In developing this work we have benefited from the support of the Global Health Section at the ISA. We were encouraged to put together two panels on African Agency and Health for the 2015 conference, which provided the space to further develop this collaborative project. We thank the panel participants for the ways their work challenged our own thinking: Sophie

Harman, Valerie Percival, Moritz Hunsmann, Peter Kingsley, Fanny Chabrol, Annamarie Bindenagel, Rene Umlauf, and Ashley Fox. We express our particular gratitude to Sophie Harman for her considered feedback on our papers and her encouragement for our project. We also extend our appreciation to our colleagues. Emma thanks her colleagues at the University of Leeds, particularly Alex Beresford, James Souter, Gordon Crawford, Ray Bush, and Michael Thomson. Amy thanks her colleagues at the University of the South for their support and encouragement, particularly Melody Crowder-Meyer, Paige Schneider, and Michael Wairungu. And she has benefited greatly from the wisdom of Gideon Byamugisha and Phoebe Kajubi.

We are also grateful for the financial resources and personal support that made the project possible. Funding for the Zambia fieldwork was provided by the Fulbright Scholar Program, a Calvin College Alumni Grant, and a Faculty Research Grant from the University of the South, while the work in Malawi was funded by the Economic and Social Research Council (ESRC) and Faculty Research Grants from Keele University and the University of Leeds. In Zambia, Sylvia Mwamba and Manenga Ndulo at the Department of Health Economics, University of Zambia; Moses Mwale and D.T. Banda at Justo Mwale Theological College; Lawrence Temfwe at Jubilee Centre; Bishop Joshua Banda at Northmead Assembly of God; John Masuwa at the Network for Zambian People Living with HIV (NZP+); Pierson Banda, HIV/AIDS Coordinator for the Reformed Church of Zambia; Gershom Kapalaula of the Zambia Network of Religious Leaders Living with or Personally Affected by HIV and AIDS; Michael Kelly of the Jesuit Centre for Theological Reflection; Angela Konayuma of the Christian Council of Zambia; and Troy Lewis of the Expanded Church Response Trust provided crucial assistance. Amy also thanks staff at the Circle of Hope AIDS clinic, clinics linked to the Centre for Infectious Disease Research in Zambia, the Christian Reformed World Relief Committee, and the Helen DeVos Christian High School, as well as Julie Limpic, the Eli Toribio family, and several NZP+ group leaders.

The work in Malawi benefited from the support of Jane Ansah, Attorney General; Kate Kainja, Minister for Women and Child Development; Anthony Kamanga, Law Commissioner; Francis Cooke, Headmaster at Kamuzu Academy; Emmanuel Fabiano, Vice Chancellor at the University of Malawi; Paul Kishindo, Director of the Centre for Social Research (CSR); and Alister Munthali with CSR. The local-level fieldwork benefited from the guidance and support of the National Coordinator of the

"Women, Girls and HIV/AIDS: Program and National Plan of Action";
the Head of Monitoring and Evaluation at the National AIDS
Commission (NAC); a representative of the Department for Nutrition,
HIV and AIDS; Program Officer for Monitoring and Evaluation at the
Malawi Network of People Living with HIV (MANET+); Assistant
Programme Manager at the National Association for People Living with
HIV and AIDS in Malawi (NAPHAM); National Coordinator at the
Coalition of Women and Girls Living with HIV/AIDS; National
Coordinator of the Malawi Network of Religious Leaders Living with
HIV and AIDS (MANERELA); Programme Coordinator of the Malawi
Network of AIDS Service Organisations (MANASO); a representative of
the National Statistics Office (NSO); and the District Coordinators for
NAPHAM in Zomba and Karonga. Emma is grateful to Al Mtenje,
Director for the Centre of Language Studies; Russell Msiska, who acted
as the facilitator and translator for the focus group discussions; and
Kondwani Klinga, who assisted in Zomba. We both thank all the partici-
pants in the key informant interviews, focus group discussions, participant
observations, and informal discussions for their time and hospitality.

And, of course, our immeasurable gratitude to our families and partners
for putting up with our late nights and early mornings at the computer,
weekends at the office, and weeks away from home doing fieldwork.
Thank you Isabel, Sophia, and Neil Patterson for your patience, love,
and desire to learn about and care for people who live far from your
small town in Tennessee. Thank you Alex Beresford for your love, support, and ability to still provide critical feedback despite the pressures of
balancing being a father to our newborn son with your own work. Thank
you Max for being such a cheerful and laid-back little man that your
mother could find the time to finish up this project while you slept.

CONTENTS

1 Dependent Agency and the AIDS Enterprise: Global
   Programs, Local Actions   1

2 Unique Opportunities in a Dynamic Aid Architecture:
   The Conditions for Agency   33

3 Performing, Extraverting, and Resisting: The Strategies
   of Dependent Agents   53

4 Complex Power on the Margins: The Implications
   of Dependent Agency   87

Bibliography   113

List of Fieldwork Data   131

Index   137

ACRONYMS

AIDS	acquired immune deficiency syndrome
ART	antiretroviral therapy
ARVs	antiretrovirals
BRICS	Brazil, Russia, India, China and South Africa
CD4	cluster of differentiation 4
CHAZ	Churches Health Association of Zambia
CBO	community-based organization
COWLHA	Coalition of Women Living with HIV and AIDS
DfID	Department for International Development
FBO	faith-based organization
FGD	focus group discussion
GDP	gross domestic product
GNI	gross national income
HBC	home-based care
HIV	human immunodeficiency virus
MANASO	Malawi Network of AIDS Service Organisations
MANET+	Malawi Network of People Living with HIV/AIDS
MoH	Ministry of Health
MOU	memorandum of understanding
MWK	Malawian kwacha
NAC Malawi	National AIDS Commission (Malawi)
NAC Zambia	National AIDS Council (Zambia)
NAPHAM	National Association for People Living with HIV and AIDS in Malawi
NGO	nongovernmental organization
NZP+	Network of Zambian People Living with HIV/AIDS
OECD	Organisation for Economic Co-operation and Development

OIG	Office of the Inspector General
PEPFAR	US President's Emergency Plan for AIDS Relief
PLHIV	person or people living with HIV
PMTCT	prevention of mother-to-child transmission
SWAp	sector-wide approach
UNAIDS	Joint United Nations Programme on HIV/AIDS
UNDP	United Nations Development Programme
USAID	United States Agency for International Development
USD	US dollar
WHO	World Health Organization
WLHIV	women living with HIV
ZMK	Zambian kwacha
ZNAN	Zambia National AIDS Network

CHAPTER 1

Dependent Agency and the AIDS Enterprise: Global Programs, Local Actions

Abstract This chapter theorizes about dependent agency and situates the concept in the Malawian and Zambian context. A condition in which people can simultaneously act and be dependent, dependent agency lies on a continuum and manifests itself to various degrees in structures of global power relations and specific environments. In Malawi and Zambia, donor competition, foreign aid uncertainty, development discourses that promote grassroots participation, global norms that define health as a human right, and the rise of the AIDS enterprise shape this global-local context. This chapter concludes by describing the research methodology.

Keywords Dependent agency · AIDS enterprise · HIV and AIDS · Africa · Malawi · Zambia

During fieldwork at a Lusaka AIDS clinic in 2011, an elderly woman approached one of the authors, wanting to "tell her story" as a person living with HIV and AIDS (PLHIV).[1] The woman was poorly dressed and quite thin; she had come to the clinic to get her monthly supply of antiretroviral treatment (ART), drugs paid for by the US President's Emergency Plan for AIDS Relief (PEPFAR). Hearing people's personal stories was common during fieldwork, though these testimonials usually were given in the context of solicited interviews. And while some researchers paid "sitting fees" to hear such stories, this author did not.

© The Author(s) 2017
E.-L. Anderson, A.S. Patterson, *Dependent Agency in the Global Health Regime*, DOI 10.1057/978-1-137-58148-8_1

1

Because the author had several appointments, there was no time to meet with the woman. The author explained the situation and went to her meetings, assuming the woman would leave. At the end of the day, the woman was still at the clinic, sitting under a tree. She approached the researcher and asked for a ride to the city center. With several clinic officials watching the exchange, the author felt uncomfortable. She knew the traffic would be terrible, but she had spent the day interviewing people about the economic needs of PLHIV. Wouldn't it be hypocritical to not give this elderly woman a ride? And she felt guilty that the woman had waited all day, even though she was pretty sure that the woman had understood that there would be no interview. Ultimately, she gave the woman a ride and a 5000 kwacha note. Only after the woman bounded from the car at the final destination did the author realize she had never even heard the woman's story (Participant observation, PLHIV-author encounter, Lusaka, May 10, 2011).

This participant observation highlights the broader themes of this volume: the various ways that individuals and communities respond to Africa's high dependency on donor health funds. We refer to these local actors as "dependent agents" and develop the concept of "dependent agency"—the condition in which these actors can simultaneously act and be dependent. Ask most people in the West about their impressions of Africa, and they will probably highlight the continent's perceived weakness and powerlessness in the international realm, its high rates of poverty and unemployment, and its deep dependence on foreign aid and commodity exports (Ayittey 1999; Englebert 2009). The continent is like the elderly woman in the Lusaka clinic: it has economic needs, some of which are met by external actors. Yet even within these broader structures of dependence, Africans show agency. They maneuver in "tight corners" in ways that demonstrate the capacity "to resist, and sometimes to deflect what appears to be their structural fate," with effects that are not inconsequential (Lonsdale 2000). For example, African states raise new issues at the UN, and some manipulate donors to gain material benefits or to avoid criticism of their authoritarian practices (Brown and Harman 2013). As an agent, the Zambian woman sought out the author, recognized the potential value of her story, decided to wait all day, changed her plans, and capitalized on the researchers' guilt and discomfort. To meet her immediate needs, the woman *acted* within the unequal and dependent structures that may undergird research, and that provide many (though not all) Western academics the resources to pay for interviews or vehicles for transportation. The observation shows that actions of dependent agents may affect those with more power and resources, a point we return to in Chapter 4. In this case, the researcher provided the woman with money and a ride, and ultimately spent hours in traffic.

This book uses the country cases of Malawi and Zambia to show how dependent agency is possible and the different forms that it takes. Agency and dependency are often seen as being mutually exclusive. Thus, on first glance the notion of dependent agency might seem slightly paradoxical. But in fact all agents are to some extent dependent, since people can only act as individuals within the social structures in which they are embedded. To be an agent necessarily means to react to some context or stimuli. Dependent agency lies on a continuum, manifesting itself to greater or lesser degrees in structures of global power relations, such as colonization, globalization, neopatrimonial governance, and aid dependence. Additionally, dependent agency shifts over time precisely because context changes with time. The exercise of dependent agency is political, for actors seek to shape the processes by which material benefits, status, or policies are gained within embedded power structures (Chabal 2014). The concept of dependent agency is particularly useful in contexts like Zambia and Malawi, because it shows that agency and dependence operate side by side even when dependence appears to be dominant.

In our study, foreign aid programs are crucial structures in which dependent agency occurs. Foreign aid plays a crucial role in the promotion of health and development in Africa. In 2013, the Organisation for Economic Co-operation and Development (OECD) countries committed USD 29 billion as aid to Africa (OECD 2013). In the case of the United States, roughly one-fourth of all foreign aid goes for health—a sector that gets more than the sectors of peace and security, humanitarian relief, or economic development (US State Department 2015). While the percentage of Africa's gross domestic product (GDP) from aid has declined for almost all countries since 1995, aid remains a crucial component of many African countries' economies. In 2013, Malawi, for example, depended on foreign aid for 40 % of its overall governmental budget and 89 % of its health budget (See *International Business Times*, November 19, 2013; Interview, MoF civil servant, Lilongwe, July 27, 2014). Foreign aid trickles down through a hierarchical chain of government agencies and international nongovernmental organizations (NGOs) to local community-based organizations (CBOs) and faith-based organizations (FBOs). This hierarchy means that local communities interact with donor organizations, sometimes acting as the agents of principals (i.e., the donors) who establish them to do the principals' work. (We discuss principal-agent issues more extensively below.) Local partners can often be highly dependent on bilateral and multilateral donors and NGOs. Susan Watkins and Ann Swidler (2013, 198) write, "NGOs come and go, and any structures they create, such as youth clubs to dramatize the dangers of AIDS or micro-finance programs to ameliorate poverty and empower women, usually evaporate when the project funding ends and the NGO departs." Aid is finite and temporal, making it crucial for local people to capitalize in timely ways on the opportunities it may provide. This situation may increase the likelihood that dependent agency manifests itself.

This book asks how people acting as individuals or as members of community organizations exert agency within these larger structures of aid dependency. We acknowledge that the potential for action is always possible, but some conditions may make it more likely that dependent agents actually act. These local responses may shape aid's effectiveness, though our central objective is not to assess the effectiveness and efficiency of foreign aid projects. We use the infusion of large amounts of donor money to address HIV and AIDS—and the subsequent retraction of that funding in 2011—as our case study. Such an examination enables us to see how Africa is "acted on" but also "actor in" global politics and develop-ment (Brown and Harman 2013). As Christopher Clapham (1996) notes with respect to African elites, it is critical to understand Africans as not simply "pawns" within an unequal configuration of global power, but as "players" with some degree of agency to invert external agendas and instrumentalize them to their own benefit. Here we focus on the players at the local level. We shed light on the dynamic interactions between actors which often occur "off stage" but which undergird macrolevel development processes.

This chapter proceeds as follows. First we introduce the scholarship on African agency. Second, we describe the global health funding con-text, through an examination of the AIDS enterprise, with its roots in HIV exceptionalism and norms on AIDS treatment. Third, we describe the cases of Malawi and Zambia, stressing their relative similarities in culture, poverty, politics, and donors' attention to AIDS. The fourth section illustrates our methodology, while the fifth outlines the themes for the rest of the book.

A Theory of African Agency

While there have always been scholars who interrogate Africans' actions as determinants of political phenomena (see Ranger 1995; Jackson and Rosberg 1984; Ottaway 1999), much of the social science literature has examined the continent through a structural lens. The modernization school assumes that development is driven by capitalism, democracy, and Western ideologies; the resulting neoliberal reforms that emerged in the 1980s sought to incorporate Africa more fully into global markets (Long 1990; Rostow 1960). Africa's political and economic development was said to rely on structures such as open trading regimes, the development of state institutions that solidify state authority, and industrial development (Huntington 1968).

When the policy prescriptions of modernization did not substantially address the continent's underdevelopment, scholars turned to neopatrimonialism as an explanation. The concept of neopatrimonailism has been used to describe a range of practices that characterize politics in Africa, including clannish behavior, so-called tribalism, patronage, cronyism, corruption, and predation (Bach and Gazibo 2012, 221). Clapham (1985, 48) defines neopatrimonalism as "a form of organization in which relationships of a broadly patrimonial type pervade a political and administrative system which is formally constructed on rational-legal lines. Officials hold positions in bureaucratic organizations with powers which are formally defined, but exercise those powers...as a form of private property." Such systems rely on the reciprocities and expectations embedded in hierarchical patron-client relations. Capturing the state becomes crucial for having the resources needed to reward clients and coopting opponents. The state has the "capacity to grant or deny access to resources and opportunities, contributing to a volatile and sometimes violent battle over who controls the 'gate'" (Beresford 2015, 229). This "gatekeeper politics" may exist alongside modern state structures, leading to the formation of hybrid systems with, on one hand, multiparty politics and the protection of some civil liberties, and on the other hand, low levels of transparency, accountability, and state capacity (Ellis 2011; Médard 1982; van de Walle 2001). According to Pierre Englebert and Kevin Dunn (2013), the resulting system undermines state capacity and long-term planning.

Some scholars have debated the usefulness of the neopatrimonialism concept, asserting that it is too formulaic to describe Africa's diverse political experiences; it does not explain state economic policies (Mkandawire 2015); it downplays how reciprocities between government officials and citizens can facilitate accountability (Pitcher et al. 2009); and it ignores the emergence of "developmental authoritarian" states like Ethiopia and Rwanda with both limited democracy and low levels of corruption (Matfess 2015). For the purposes of our work, the concept minimizes African agency and the multiple ways that actors react to their contexts. In the model, state actors become trapped by the patronage structures that undergird political parties, legislatures, and bureaucracies and that hamper creative and autonomous actions (Englebert and Dunn 2013; Wrong 2010). "Individual choices are ultimately determined... by the ubiquitous logic of neopatrimonialism.... and social actors do what they do reflexively, or even compulsively" (Mwandawire 2015, 598). In this work, we do not engage the debates over the accuracy of the neopatrimonial portrayal of African politics. In our two case studies—Malawi and Zambia—some aspects of patronage, reciprocal obligations, and gatekeeper politics exist, as the following chapters indicate. But they are not solely determinant of how our dependent agents react to donor projects on AIDS at the local level. We recognize both the existence of neopatrimonial structures and the ability of individuals to maneuver around, reinterpret, utilize, and at times, be constrained by these structures.

Other theoretical perspectives also view the continent through a structural lens. Dependency scholars argue that the global economic system exploits Africa, through unequal trade structures and unrepresentative international financial institutions (Evans 1979). Similarly, realist theory highlights how Africa lacks the military might, geostrategic importance, and economic resources needed to be a player in global power shifts (Dunn and Shaw 2001). As a result, Africa's hard power weakness limits its global influence. And development studies often assert that Africa's aid dependence allows donors to set agendas and prioritize particular issues with little input from recipient states or their populations (Jalali 2013).

All of these structural approaches have a tendency to downplay agentic behavior embedded within those structures (Wendt 1987) and to provide "determinist, linear and externalist views of social change" (Long 1990, 6). They also prioritize the state as an actor by ignoring nonstate actors like political parties, churches, or community groups, and they typically focus on more powerful Western players as actors in Africa. In response, we acknowledge that social change is a nonlinear, messy process, and, like Will Reno (1998) who shows that linkages between multinational corporations and rebel movements in West Africa can undermine the state, we see that nonstate actors are crucial in political change and development processes. Nonstate actors also may develop their own goals, autonomy, and identities (Barnett and Finnemore 2004). Drawing upon Long (1990, 6), we call for an "actor-oriented" approach to African political and socioeconomic development which does not ignore the state and global structures but which moves beyond them to understand "the self-organising practices of those inhabiting, experiencing and transforming the contours and details of social landscape."

As a more specifically actor-oriented approach, principal-agent theory seeks to understand how institutions function and sometimes, fail. Rooted in rationalist approaches that view actors as central protagonists who calculate costs and benefits, the theory examines the relationships that emerge when principals delegate authority to agents to achieve a certain function on the principals' behalf (Kassim and Menon 2003). The theory highlights how principals and agents may have different objectives, and how this may result in agents' shirking duties or developing their own tasks. While principal-agent theory sheds some light on the types of relationships we explore (and we allude to those insights below), the theory faces limitations in the study of community-based development projects. First, it assumes that principals establish agents (e.g., the idea that states establish international organizations). While principals like donors do sometimes set up local development organizations to be their agents, it is more often the case that principals seek to partner with already existing organizations. Second, the model assumes that principals have some control over agents through institutional design. Yet in the case of many grassroots development organizations, there are no formalized institutional rules: membership is fluid, decision-making processes are obtuse (even if they are codified), and ramifications for not meeting project requirements are unclear (Patterson 2003). Donor–local agent relationships are often personalized and dynamic (Krause 2014). Finally, the theory defines agents to be institutions: organizations, groups, firms, and associations. Yet we recognize that agents are also individuals.

We stress that agency is human initiative in thought or action; it embodies intentional acts taken on behalf of someone (even if that someone is the individual) (Onuf 2003). The intentions prior to the act are not crucial to agency; instead, it is the ability to act that matters (Giddens 1984, 1–16). Agency may only be recognized in hindsight, after the action or word is performed. Agents often have an element of creativity. They may delve into a repertoire of symbols, cultural practices, actions, and/or vocabularies to shape messages, to convey opinions, and to challenge or agree with prevailing power structures (Frueh 2013). James C. Scott (1990), for example, illustrates how subordinate groups in society such as slaves, prisoners, serfs, and employees may use gossip, foot-dragging, and derogatory stories to resist the structures and ideologies of domination that surround them. The concept of agency gives the individual actor capacity to "devise ways of coping with life, even under the most extreme forms of coercion" (Long 1990, 8). Actors are "knowledgeable" and "capable," though they work within contexts of uncertainty. Just like the Zambian woman in the introduction to this chapter, they learn, solve problems, and observe how others react to them; they actively engage in "constructing their own social worlds" (Long 1990, 8). These are dynamic processes; agency is a "process of becoming rather than a state of being: agency as promise rather than premise" (Chabal et al. 2007, 3).

The focus on agency "does not necessarily lead away from grand political, even structural, narratives, full of 'big why explanations'" (Long 1990, 15). Instead, it helps us to better understand how those "big why explanations" work. As John Lonsdale (2000, 5) recognizes, local case studies of the "linkages between the personal, the social, and the political, can in fact suggest answers to 'the big why questions' of larger historical process." We learn how "these processes are in real life perceived, and contingently acted upon, by historically knowledgeable human agents." Agency itself is a political phenomenon—constantly negotiated between structures and individual actions. Our dependent agents interface with the structures of foreign aid, as well as the cultural, political, and economic contexts of Malawi and Zambia (see below and Chapter 2). We stress two points about the structure–agency linkage. First, structures may provide some room in which agents maneuver: they create material opportunities, spread ideologies, or distribute resources for agents (Brown and Harman 2013, 3). Second, agency and structures are "mutually constituting" (Brown 2012, 1890); structures may be changed, even if only at the margins. They are not static or immutable. For local agents, these small changes are not inconsequential. It is in these moments that our agents illustrate power. Chapter 4 highlights how dependent agents can cause donors to rethink projects or to limit demands in specific contexts.

The concept of dependent agency recognizes that actors have interests, from gaining access to material goods, to advancing normative ideals, to investing in relations that will ensure their long-term security

(Hyden 1980). Agents' goals may be multiple and dynamic, and they may be rooted in cultural identities and ideologies (see Finnemore and Sikkink 1998). In short, dependent agency has a purpose (Brown and Harman 2013, 7). Agents' objectives may inform the words and actions they use. For example, agents with a normative agenda may emphasize the donor-accepted norm of a right to health in their speech acts with donors. Recognizing the interests involved in dependent agency does not mean that we are taking a rationalist approach, because we also recognize that agents may have competing objectives or not even be able to recognize or articulate their interests.

CONDITIONS FOR AND STRATEGIES OF DEPENDENT AGENTS

When is dependent agency possible and what does it look like? Chapters 2 and 3 will specifically address these questions in the context of the AIDS enterprise and shifts in donor attention in Malawi and Zambia. Here we outline a theory of conditions and provide examples of agentic strategies. We do not assert that each condition is necessary, and we do not claim that this list is exhaustive. Agency does not happen all of the time and it does not occur in a vacuum. We recognize that agency is often practiced through what Scott (1990, 14) terms "hidden transcripts," or the behind-the-scenes words and deeds of both the dominant and subordinate parties in unequal relationships. In this analysis, we focus on the hidden transcripts of the dependent agents not donors. The HIV "crisis" with its exceptional donor response and shift in donor funding sheds light on the discrepancy between the public and the hidden transcripts. It also presents an opportunity to examine the structures of power previously accepted as the status quo and the agency of the seemingly powerless (Scott 1990, 16).

The first set of conditions for dependent agency relates to the multitude of donors, each with competing and dynamic programs (Chinsinga 2007). The foreign aid field has innumerable actors: the 29 states in the Development Assistance Committee of OECD, some of the BRICS countries, some Middle Eastern states, and hundreds of international NGOs and FBOs. These actors partner with local groups, and in countries where donors prefer to work (because of prior history, strategic reasons, shared language and/or religion, or geographic proximity), local communities can be inundated with donor projects (Krause 2014). When dependent agents have choices between donor partners, they have more opportunities to autonomously advance their own interests. During the cold war, for example, African state leaders played one superpower off of the other to get foreign aid (Brown 2012). More recently, China's role as an aid provider and trade partner has given African leaders similar opportunities (Taylor 2009). Recent interest in Malawi from the Chinese provides opportunities for leverage for the Ministry of Health (MoH) at a time when there has been a retraction of support from the traditional donors (Interview, MoH civil servant, Lilongwe, June 28, 2014). At the local level, when multiple NGOs decide to work in the same community, participants may float between groups, "shopping around" to see where they can get the best benefits (Interview, PLHIV, Lusaka, May 4, 2011).

Donors' "preferences heterogeneity" in aid projects may provide political space for agency (Hawkins et al. 2006). Donors differ on methods and priorities: Canada often gives direct budgetary aid, while the United States gives funds primarily to American NGOs who then partner with indigenous groups. China supports infrastructure projects through loans, while the European Union focuses on human capacity building (Taylor 2009). While the lack of unity in approaches and requirements could decrease the agency of poor recipients (van der Veen 2011), this need not always be the case. Instead, as donors bicker among themselves, they may become distracted, giving dependent agents considerable discretion in and space for agency.

As a dynamic arena, the foreign aid field provides "uncertain moments" on which dependent agents might capitalize. Donor contributions rise and fall with the "swinging pendulum" of shifting political priorities, and donors become more (or less) interested in certain areas having issues (Lee 2004). Dynamism is evident in AIDS programs: donor funding increased from USD 200 million in 1996 to roughly USD 8.6 billion in 2014 (Kaiser Family Foundation 2015b). In Chapter 2, we draw attention to the particularities of the shifts in AIDS funding in Malawi and Zambia from 2009—changes rooted in the global financial crisis, deteriorating donor relations, and concerns surrounding accountability for donor funds. Over the years, donors have also changed their emphases: unlike in the early days of the pandemic, they now stress ART adherence and HIV prevention over care and support for PLHIV. In periods when new programs are developing or changing, dependent agents have more "wiggle room" to act.

If the dynamic and varied approaches of multiple donors create opportunities for agency, what strategies might dependent agents use? We focus on three in this volume: performances of compliance, extraversion, and resistance. The first is performances of compliance, in which local actors echo the "official story" of the rhetoric, symbols, structures, and ideologies of donors in order to gain resources or representation. For example, PLHIV may use the jargon of AIDS programs (e.g., "living positively") and they may disclose their HIV status publicly in order to appeal to donors. Some, like the Zambian woman in the introduction of this chapter, may want to tell their personal histories, because donors have emphasized the cathartic importance of such experiences (Nguyen 2010; Benton 2015). Others may exaggerate their exuberance about donor-initiated projects in order to please donors (Scott 1990, 67, 139). There may be widespread uptake of certain practices that at least appear to "make everyone happy," with a key example being embrace of and demand for training sessions (Watkins and Swidler 2013, 207). In a sense, by using these "public transcripts" (Scott 1990), local people may seem to be reinforcing the structures of power, inequality, and dependence embedded in foreign aid. They may appear to be "active accomplices to their own subordination" (Long 1990, 14). Yet the reality is more complex. These performances demonstrate local agents' desire to never burn bridges, for one never knows when someone may need the support of a powerful patron such as a donor or its local emissaries (Ferguson 2013; Hyden 1980). Better to pretend excitement than to anger an external agent. As the Wolof proverb asserts, *"Fen wuy defar moo gën dàgg guy yaq."* (Lies that build are better than truths that destroy.) Yet these performances are not static and our empirical material collected from 2005 until 2014 enables us to examine how this process changes over time. Chapter 3 shows that in the process of "acting the mask," the performer's face may grow to fit the mask. The performer may come to believe the performance, and thus, the performance may no longer serve to resist the dominant party or to gain resources from it (Scott 1990, 9–10).

In addition, if the actions of powerful partners (in our case, donors) do not resonate with the public transcript, dependent agents may charge hypocrisy. After all, the powerful too are required to act in certain ways, and performances of the dominant are necessary to support their claims to legitimacy (Scott 1990, 10). The need for legitimacy can provide leverage for the seemingly powerless partner. At the international level, Martha Finnemore (2009) shows that the United States has been criticized as hypocritical when it does not live up to its rhetoric on human rights or democracy. If the powerful care about their reputations (and reputations bring legitimacy, which makes it easier to accomplish rule), they may react to such charges, though reactions may not always mean changing policies.

Much of the public transcript about foreign aid is normative (e.g., "saving lives," "building human capabilities," or "combatting inequalities"). This normative agenda is compounded by the West's history of oppression with Africa. Donors, therefore, may be particularly sensitive to charges of hypocrisy (van de Walle 2001). In addition, the emphasis that FBOs put on charity, human dignity, and compassion may make them susceptible. The public transcript surrounding aid—that donors are powerful but benevolent—may be challenged if donors' actions are not perceived to be benevolent. While very few dependent agents at the local level would openly charge a donor with hypocrisy, they may use rhetoric that gently reminds the donor of its commitment to globally accepted human rights norms or religious tenets of compassion. As they indirectly charge hypocrisy, dependent agents may lead to subtle redefinitions of the public transcript. For example, Christian compassion may be defined to include meeting the immediate needs of PLHIV not just fostering sustainable projects (see Scherz 2014). Even the possibility that a dependent agent could utilize hypocrisy may empower the weak. For example, Tanzanian health officials recognize that donors will not cut funding for ART to Africans already on treatment, because the deaths that result would make Western policymakers vulnerable to charges of heartlessness in the media and among activists. This realization enables Tanzanian officials to limit state spending on ART and the AIDS response (Hunsmann 2015).

More broadly, the ideologies that undergird development projects may provide space for local agency (Long 1990). Concepts like "participation" and "targeting the poor" call for local involvement, and methodologies such as participatory action research require that local individuals help to build development programs (Chambers 1997). Donors emphasize sustainability, or giving people the skills needed to continue projects once the donor is gone (Scherz 2014). They foster local capacity by teaching local people budgeting, report writing, planning, and management techniques. When donors provide trainings or give start-up capital or inputs, they seek to empower community members. And local populations, using the donor's rhetoric of empowerment, may request these opportunities, because trainings bring skills and they include material incentives like meals, transport fees, and per diems (Smith 2003). While the "sustainability doctrine" and the practices that emerge from it may theoretically empower, Ann Swidler and Susan Watkins (2009) demonstrate that trained volunteers lose the opportunity to earn income, making it difficult for them to volunteer indefinitely. Illustrating their agency, some volunteers may quit,

an action that necessitates training more volunteers. Donors' local empowerment may create agents who do not promote donors' goals, the classic
principal-agent problem. People may become empowered though not
necessarily in the ways that were intended; instead they may learn to better
navigate and compete for aid resources. In the long term, empowerment
"run[s] counter to the idea of makeability and, therefore, counter to inter-
ventionist paradigms that assume the possibility of guided if not 'mechan-
ical' transformations of social realities" (De Bruijn et al. 2007, 15).

The second strategy we examine is extraversion. As Jean-François
Bayart (2000) argues, Africa's historical embeddedness in the international arena and the ways that external actors perceive the continent and
its people shape opportunities for agency. Despite the emergence of an
"Africa rising" rhetoric (see Economist 2013), the prevailing view of
Africa is that the continent is mired in poverty and pervasive violent
conflict, economically dependent, technologically backward, and disease-
ridden (Chabal et al. 2007, 1). Dependent agents may emphasize these
portrayals in order to gain benefits, with a "deliberate recourse to the
strategy of extraversion, mobilizing resources derived from their (possibly
unequal) relationship with the external environment" (Bayart 2000, 218).
The international environment becomes a "major resource in the process
of political centralization and economic accumulation," because it allows
African actors to gain rents (Bayart 2000, 219). Extraversion is a conscious
strategy, with African elites "doing everything they can" to encourage
their own dependence and to highlight their problems (Ellis 2011, 6).
Witness, for example, Liberian President Ellen Sirleaf Johnson's public
pleas for help during the 2014–2015 West Africa Ebola epidemic (*New
York Times*, September 12, 2014). While the affected countries in West
Africa needed resources, the West's willingness to provide them was
rooted in perceptions of Africa as the primitive arena from which deadly
diseases originate (Wilkinson and Leach 2014). Research on Sierra Leone
reveals how the crisis situation could be used as leverage for attracting
support and how the influx of resources provided lucrative opportunities
for rent seeking and corruption (Anderson and Beresford 2016).

Extraversion extends beyond political elites since actors at multiple
levels manipulate their situations in order to get access to resources.
Research in Tanzania and Kenya, for example, examines how in
response to economic and political liberalization groups extravert
their cultural distinctiveness—"becoming indigenous peoples"—in
order to mobilize resources and moral, political, and legal advantage

(Igoe 2006; Lynch 2012, 8; Hodgson 2011). Where HIV has been treated as an exceptional issue that attracts unprecedented levels of funding as compared to other health issues, it provides new avenues for extraversion, including through people presenting themselves as HIV positive—"becoming HIV positive peoples"—even if they are not, so that they may access resources and gain other forms of leverage (Anderson 2015, 143–144; Benton 2015, 53–55).

As a "mode of action," extraversion is a dynamic process that state and nonstate actors embrace and that stresses Africa's dependence on the West in conjunction with the West's dependence on Africa (Bayart 2000, 218; see also; Burchardt 2013). Donors' need for resources, strategic allies, and arenas in which to promote their ideologies has enabled Africa to benefit (Peiffer and Englebert 2012). Stephen Ellis (2011, 6, 33) writes that "dependency has been a joint venture" and that "the tens of thousands of Westerners, ranging from sandal-wearing volunteers through to the highly paid consultants found in five-star hotels, would have to look for a new line of work if Africa stopped needing aid." The West's own dependence on Africa's perceived poverty and weakness and the West's willingness to go along with extraversion may result in what James Ferguson (1994) calls the "anti-politics machine," or emphasis on the technical nature of development processes that does not challenge the deeper issues of dependency, inequalities, or underrepresentation that underscore underdevelopment. Extraversion may be a "conservative" strategy for dependent agents and their Western supporters.

The final strategy we explore is what Scott terms "resistance below the line," or disguised resistance to structures of domination without which the "loud form of public resistance" (or actions outside of the proverbial "line") is impossible (Scott 1990, 198–199). These behind-the-scenes actions of the subordinate are not just posing; they are an arena of practice, one that is not necessarily benign to the processes and powers of the dominant actors. "The discourse of the hidden transcript does not merely shed light on behavior or explain it; it helps to constitute that behavior" (Scott 1990, 189; see also 185–187). In this resistance, the subordinate moves between "the world of the master and the offstage world of subordinates" (Scott 1990, 191). In the context of our work, we note various types of resistance below the line: foot-dragging, stretching the rules, using euphemisms, and redefining the issue. For example, dependent agents may be slow to meet project requirements, particularly if they think there may be other donor opportunities. If multiple donors present what locals see as onerous demands (from report writing to monthly meetings), dependent agents might claim confusion as an excuse for slow (or nonexistent) action. They also may capitalize on uncertainties in donor programs to redefine the issue; that is, they may remake the issue to fit donors' new visions for aid or bring new interpretations to rules to benefit their own agendas (Interview, NGO official, July 4, 2014). For example, groups that used to focus solely on palliative home-based care (HBC) for PLHIV may now call themselves HIV prevention groups to meet donors' increased interest in HIV prevention.

In all three strategies, we see a role for brokers, whose presence is possible because donors depend on intermediaries who link them to local communities: they need people who can introduce, translate, guide, and support their efforts. But local communities need these brokers too, since they understand the donor world and can help community members to interpret it. Acting as a broker is an entrepreneurial strategy; these dependent agents recognize the donors' needs, the ways to meet those needs, and the potential benefits that they may personally gain as brokers. Because brokers can translate the interactions between donors and the community, they can frame and reframe issues to meet their own objectives (Lewis and Mosse 2006, 15). They often specialize in acquiring, controlling, and redistributing development revenues. They too learn the performances required of them to establish their own legitimacy and differentiate themselves from the "backward masses," using the required narratives of "harmful cultural practices" and "foolish villagers" to set themselves apart (Watkins and Swidler 2013, 201; Englund 2006). "Brokers all up and down the [AIDS enterprise] hierarchy play the role of 'authentic African' for foreign visitors to embrace" (Watkins and Swidler 2013, 201). Those who are relatively powerful at the local level (including local authorities and NGO workers) employ tactics to access and control the limited resources and opportunities that are available (see Kingsley 2014).

Brokers became a crucial part of the AIDS enterprise, which we discuss below. As Watkins and Swidler (2013, 200–201) consider:

As the AIDS industry grew, participating NGOs could offer opportunities for formal employment outside of government. This contributed to expanding the middle class and enhancing the perceived value of education. In Malawi there is now a clearly understood hierarchy of career possibilities based on educational credentials, from a volunteer in a small village community-based organization (CBO), appealing to youths with secondary education and no other hope for escaping village life, to a Ph.D. in a UN agency in Lilongwe with a salary large enough to provide first-world health care for his or her family and first-world education for his or her children.

As AIDS brought new opportunities, brokers developed multiple motivations for their actions that extend beyond solely acquiring material benefits. Watkins and Swidler (2013, 201) continue, "Brokers may also have other aspirations: to maintain their status in the local community, to manage the support of myriad relatives and other dependents, to cultivate local networks, to attain the next-higher educational credential." They also may have few incentives to engage with the politics of development since they are beneficiaries of the system, thus contributing to the conservative nature of development processes. But because foreign aid conditions are dynamic, brokers' situation is precarious. They remain "marginal and vulnerable figure[s] located between fault lines and connection points within complex systems and relationships" (Lewis and Mosse 2006, 12).

It is important to recognize that the aforementioned conditions and strategies are situated in a "given social site" (Scott 1990, 14), and dependent agents may tie their actions to cultural expectations and practices (Long 1990). Rituals related to gender, caste, religion, ethnicity, or age may provide avenues by which agency is practiced or idioms around which agency may be defined. The institutions associated with these practices such as churches, mosques, women's clubs, school yards, and social gatherings may be physical spaces in which hidden transcripts flourish (Nepstad 2011; Scott 1990). Because donors often do not understand these spaces and practices, there is little recrimination when agency and alternative visions develop within them. On the issue of AIDS, for example, such spaces have allowed some Pentecostal churches to design HIV prevention programs that contradict those supported by many public health officials (Gusman 2009).

In summary, agency reflects human initiative, intentionally manifested in words and actions in order to achieve an objective. The conditions under which agency may emerge are numerous, and may include uncertain dynamic aid structures that result from donors who lack unity in their approaches. Public transcripts provide opportunities for performances of compliance and/or claims of hypocrisy, both strategies that enable agents to demand benefits and redefine issues. And donors' own rhetoric, symbols, and ideologies may create possibilities for agency. All of these conditions rely on Africa's relationship with global partners who often interact with the continent using simplistic narratives. Strategies of performances of compliance, extraversion, and resistance below the line are some of the ways agency manifests itself.

THE AIDS ENTERPRISE

Our dependent agents are situated in a context with a legacy of high global attention to AIDS in Africa. This attention has resulted in what Watkins and Swidler (2013) term the "AIDS enterprise," a hierarchy of AIDS-related organizations that reaches from bilateral and multilateral donors to local community organizations. At each level, donors may engage with local partners, other donors, or NGOs; thus money "flows chaotically both downward and sideways" (Watkins and Swidler 2013, 199). The enterprise includes large-scale donor efforts like PEPFAR and the Global Fund for AIDS, Tuberculosis and Malaria (Global Fund), two funding mechanisms which require donors to back up rhetoric on AIDS (and particularly, AIDS treatment) with resources. It includes efforts by private foundations, like the Clinton Health Access Initiative which pools low-income states' purchasing power so they may negotiate for the lowest price on generic AIDS drugs (Kapstein and Busby 2013). Complete with an organizational machinery, the AIDS enterprise has rules for action (e.g., the importance of monitoring and evaluation) and a particular jargon (e.g., PLHIV are referred to as "clients" not "patients"). It requires particular state structures such as government AIDS commissions and Country Coordinating Mechanisms (which apply for and manage Global Fund grants). And because of the disease's pervasive effects on individuals, communities, and societies, it demands a multisectoral approach: HIV care, treatment, support, and prevention programs are embedded in multiple ministries (Putzel 2004).

The most notable aspect of the AIDS enterprise is its sizeable amount of funding: the disease has attracted global commitments and resources on an unprecedented level as compared to other health concerns (see Smith and Whiteside 2010; Nguyen 2010, 13). In 2014, donors gave over USD 8.6 billion for the AIDS response (Dionne et al. 2013; Kaiser Family Foundation 2015b). This funding is in reaction to Africa's high HIV prevalence: 24 million Africans were HIV positive and 1.1 million died from AIDS in 2013 (UNAIDS 2014). Donor AIDS funding has been dynamic: the biggest increase occurred between 2001 (USD 1.2 billion) and 2008 (USD 7.8 billion). But because of the global financial crisis of

2008, funding stagnated in 2009 and then decreased to below 2008 levels until 2013. In that year, funding increased to USD 8.5 billion, but levels in 2014 were only marginally higher (at USD 8.6 billion). In 2014, funding from 9 of 14 donor governments declined, while funding from the United States and Germany remained flat (Kaiser Family Foundation 2015b). These aggregate level changes in funding mask individual country experiences such as cuts in donor funding like Zambia and Malawi faced in 2011. Yet even despite the recent stagnation in funding, donors' continued attention to AIDS cannot be denied.

The AIDS enterprise is rooted in the portrayal of HIV and AIDS as "an unprecedented emergency with global consequences" and an exceptional health condition (Watkins and Swidler 2013, 198). In 2005, then director of UNAIDS Peter Piot said, "This pandemic is exceptional because there is no plateau in sight, exceptional because of the severity and longevity of its impact, and exceptional because of the special challenges it poses to effective public action" (Benton 2015, x). HIV exceptionalism has led to vertical (disease-specific) programs in which AIDS is treated differently from other diseases. HIV exceptionality led to the aforementioned new policy and health structures, and it drove donors to devote high levels of attention to AIDS in countries with low (and stable) HIV rates and with health challenges that affected more people than HIV does (Benton 2015).

HIV exceptionalism has been criticized on numerous levels. Emergency responses to the exceptional challenges HIV poses are at odds with dealing with health issues such as HIV as "long wave" events (Barnett and Prinns 2006, 360). Roger England (2007) asserts that the attention to AIDS has not led to a measurable decline in HIV infections. AIDS funding may have displaced spending on other health issues, though these effects may have not been apparent in the mid-2000s because of the overall increase in global health spending (Shiffman 2008). Even though AIDS advocates assert that money spent on AIDS benefits many health issues, Shiffman et al. (2009) dispute that assertion. AIDS funding has only had a marginal impact on infectious disease control and no effect on health system strengthening or population and reproductive health. Karen Grépin (2012) illustrates that AIDS funding has had mixed results, crowding out childhood immunization efforts in countries with few health care providers but increasing some maternal health services. In Malawi, the health sector has become warped by the "brain drain" of expertise from other areas of health as practitioners shift to work on HIV because it is more lucrative (Interview, MoH civil servant, Lilongwe, July 28, 2014). So too, local development dynamics have changed: local organizations that focus on AIDS have benefitted, leaving NGOs that work on education and agriculture with less funding and staffing challenges (Morfit 2011). In his work on West Africa, Vinh-Kim Nguyen (2010, 177, 186) highlights the "logic of triage," which includes the bundling of services for PLHIV. This "government-by-exception" brings with it new categories of belonging, new ways of arbitrating life and death, and new forms of exception and exclusion. Community programs that focus solely on AIDS may divide members of poor communities along sero-status lines (Patterson 2015; Anderson 2015, 144; Boesten 2011).

Additionally, the AIDS enterprise emerged from norms, or socially constructed expectations for "standard[s] of appropriate behavior for actors with a given identity" (Finnemore and Sikkink 1998, 891). States which are concerned about how other states perceive them often feel social pressure to adopt and implement norms. Global health governance has embodied several contentious norms, such as the expectation that states should promote population health ("right to health" or the "right to primary health care") and the expectation that states should report contagious disease outbreaks under the International Health Regulations (Davies et al. 2015; Youde 2008). Some scholars assert that states have accepted the norm of access to ART, because they have created the aforementioned programs to fund medications for millions of PLHIV (Kapstein and Busby 2013; Youde 2008).

The asserted norm of access to ART is rooted in two broad ideational trajectories. The first is the rhetoric of human rights. As "timeless expressions of fundamental entitlements of the human condition," human rights reflect the value of human dignity, the desire for justice, the protection from suffering, and equal protection of all from discrimination (Nguyen-Krug and Hogerzeil 2006). Since the early days of the AIDS response, activists and health experts have framed action against AIDS in terms of human rights, recognizing that violations of socioeconomic and political rights make individuals more vulnerable to HIV infection and that AIDS, because of its lethality and associated stigma, undermines PLHIV's basic right to life, health, work, family, and education. As a result, the protection of human rights, including the right of PLHIV to participate in decision-making and to not be discriminated against in all walks of life, is essential (Mann 1999). Framing ART access in the larger context of human rights has enabled activists to draw on crucial normative expectations about protection of human life, nondiscrimination, and access to resources that promote human capabilities, all of which have been codified in human rights treaties such as the Universal Declaration of Human Rights, the Alma Ata Declaration, and the Convention of the Rights of the Child (Reubi 2011; Olesen 2006).

The second ideational trajectory is faith-based approaches to health, suffering, and death. While religious individuals and institutions have been criticized for their stigmatizing actions and rhetoric against PLHIV (Patterson 2013), in reality faith-based approaches have been heterogeneous. Religious leaders in Africa and the West have used sacred texts to emphasize compassion, care, and alleviation of suffering to support the expansion of ART access. For example, Muslim leaders in Nigeria supported ART access, because "God has never made a disease for which He has not also sent its medicine" (Tocco 2010). In Zambia, church leaders and FBO officials spoke of the need to show God's love to others by providing medications: "Jesus said to care for the 'least of these', the sick, the widows, and the hungry. That means helping them get medicine" (Interview, FBO official, Lusaka, August 15, 2007).

States do not accept all norms, but they are more likely to accept a norm if it embodies protection of innocent groups from bodily harm and legal equality of opportunity (Finnemore and Sikkink 1998). The norm of access to AIDS treatment fits these conditions, particularly when activists, celebrities, and politicians emphasized the deaths of children and women in their advocacy for universal ART access (Kapstein and Busby 2013). The norm appeared to be widely accepted when all UN member-states signed the 2001 Declaration of Commitment which explicitly called for universal access, when the World Health Organization (WHO) endorsed the specific goal of placing three million PLHIV who needed ART on medication by 2005, and when world leaders such as US President George W. Bush promoted access to AIDS medications (Youde 2008; Bush 2003). As a result, by 2015, 15 million people (or 41 % of those who needed ART) could access AIDS medications. In 2002, only one million PLHIV globally (and only 300,000 PLHIV in low and middle-income countries) had ART access. In Africa, the number of PLHIV on ART has expanded from under 100,000 in 2002 to over 10.7 million in 2015; in 2014, 43 % of PLHIV in sub-Saharan Africa who needed the medications could access them (UNAIDS 2015; WHO, UNICEF, and UNAIDS 2013).

We acknowledge that the norm of universal access to ART is threatened by the slowdown in AIDS funding, AIDS fatigue among donors and citizens in the West and Africa, and the fact that the number of PLHIV needing ART continues to increase as PLHIV currently on ART live longer and as newly tested PLHIV are urged to begin treatment before symptoms emerge (Kaiser Family Foundation 2015a; *Science Speaks*, July 19, 2015). Despite these challenges, the norm's existence provides the opportunity for our dependent agents to use the expectation that donor states should provide ART to advance their objectives. The legitimacy of those who agreed to the norm can be questioned if they do not live up to its expectations. Legitimacy shapes the credibility of future commitments and ultimately, the ability of powerful donors to get support for and local participation in their development agendas. Such a consideration is relevant since the development enterprise's neoliberal focus relies heavily on local mobilization and individual initiative (Ferguson 2010; Scherz 2014; Anderson 2015; Harvey 2005).

In this volume, we focus on how local organizations react to the AIDS enterprise: its programs, its multiple actors and layers, its embedded norms, its unanticipated consequences, and its dynamism, particularly in terms of donors' shift in attention from AIDS by 2011. These organizations include support groups for PLHIV; caregiving groups that assist PLHIV or AIDS orphans; local organizations that provide HIV education; and community clinics that test for HIV and provide ART. Some of these groups are secular and others are faith-based. While some existed before donors were concerned about AIDS, many others emerged with donors' heightened attention to the disease. They have all in some way benefited from the AIDS enterprise, though they sometimes do not support some of its aspects, such as donors' desire for HIV disclosure. Some discount the idea that HIV deserves exceptional attention and point to other development concerns beyond AIDS (see Dionne 2012). Our investigation of dependent agency helps us to understand how individuals and community groups both benefit from and challenge the AIDS enterprise.

THE COUNTRY CASES

We have chosen two countries with many similarities in order to confirm patterns we see in local agency. Both share many historical, cultural, and political experiences, as well as high rates of poverty and deep incorporation into the AIDS enterprise, and both were British colonies that gained independence in 1964. Zambia is larger geographically and is more sparsely populated, with 15.5 million people compared to Malawi with 17.9 million (World Bank 2015a, b). Both have Christian majorities, though Malawi has a more sizeable Muslim minority (around 12 % of the population) than Zambia does (around 3 %) (CIA 2015a, b). While mainline Protestants and Catholics historically dominated each country, Pentecostalism is spreading rapidly (Cheyeka 2009). Both countries are ethnically diverse. In Zambia, no ethnic group has sufficient numbers to dominate politics; parties tend to be cross-ethnic, and several ethnic groups (such as the Chewa and Tumbuka) consider themselves political allies. In Malawi, the Chewas and Tumbukas are relatively large groups with antagonistic relations. Political parties are formed along ethnic lines and because the Chewa are more numerous (roughly one-third of the population), they have more opportunities to shape political outcomes (Posner 2004).

Both countries are highly dependent on foreign aid. In 2011, 40 % of the Malawian government's overall budget came from external resources and 40 % of that aid came from the United Kingdom (Interview, MoF civil servant, Lilongwe, June 26, 2014; *International Business Times*, November 19, 2013). In Zambia, the percentage was 28.5 % (World Bank 2014). In both countries, the health sector is highly dependent on external funds because of the governments' limited tax base. In Malawi, the MoH receives 89 % of its funding from external resources (again, 40 % of which was from DfID). In Zambia, this percentage was 55 % in 2009 (*IRIN News*, May 27, 2009). This reliance on donors was even more apparent in terms of AIDS: as a PEPFAR focus country, 84 % of Zambia's AIDS funding came from PEPFAR, 5 % from multilateral donors, and the rest from government and private sources (Zambia NAC 2014, 42). In Malawi, 84 % of the AIDS funding came from development partners, 14 % from government, and 2 % from private sources (GoM 2015, 52). Zambia received USD 1.4 billion from PEPFAR between 2004 and 2014, while Malawi was awarded USD 351 million between 2003 and 2015 (PEPFAR 2014, 2015). The Global Fund has granted Zambia USD 662 million, while it has provided Malawi with USD 705 million (Global Fund 2015a, b). This funding supported hundreds of treatment, care, and prevention efforts.

Both countries are highly reliant on exports: Zambia on copper and Malawi on agriculture (particularly burley tobacco), and both are vulnerable to exogenous economic shocks. Yet, Zambia had fared better until 2015 because of the high price of copper on the global market (and high demand for that copper from China, the country's largest trading partner), as well as economic diversification into an increasingly productive agricultural sector. As a result, the country had annual growth rates of roughly

6 % each year between 2003 and 2015, and a low inflation rate of roughly 7 %. Its gross national income (GNI) per capita in 2014 was USD 1760 (World Bank 2015b). Zambia also weathered the global financial crisis of 2008–2009 relatively well, only experiencing a short-term drop in trade, remittances, and foreign investments in 2009 (Ndulo et al. 2010). Growth rates had returned by 2010. However, by mid-2015, the global price of copper had dropped over 20 %, leading to a decline in the kwacha (ZMK), economists to slash the country's predicted growth rate to 3 % for 2016, unemployment to grow rapidly, and food prices to increase by over 20 % (AfDB 2015; *The Globe and Mail*, October 26, 2015).

In 2011 and 2012, Malawi experienced the worst economic crisis since independence; past economic gains were undermined by the large trade deficit and an overvalued fixed exchange rate. The result was acute shortages of fuel and electricity blackouts that impinged on the private sector, as well as a foreign exchange crunch (DfID 2012b, 2). This crisis was compounded by deteriorating diplomatic relations under the then government of President Bingu wa Mutharika, as indicated in Chapter 2. In anticipation of reduced external support, the government introduced taxes on water, bread, milk, and meat as part of the "zero-deficit" austerity budget (see Wroe 2012). By 2012, economic growth slowed to 2.1 % (AfDB 2014); rising costs of living and increased unemployment levels negatively impacted the poorest in society. Although economic growth reached 5.7 % in 2014 (driven largely by agriculture), inflation was 24.1 % because of the continued depreciation of the kwacha (MWK) and withdrawal of donor budgetary support (AfDB 2014). In 2014, Malawi remained among the poorest countries in the world with a GNI of USD 240 (World Bank 2015a).

Most crucial for our study—since we focus on local responses to donor dependence—is the fact that both countries have high rates of poverty in the communities where we conducted our research. Zambia experienced a deep economic depression during the 1990s, when the price of copper plummeted and copper mines were privatized. Redundant miners moved from middle-class areas of the Copperbelt to slum communities in Ndola, Kitwe, and Lusaka (Ferguson 1999). The economic stagnation drove farmers to cities, increasing urban problems and inequalities. As of 2014, 40 % of Zambians lived in urban areas, where over 70 % of people work in the informal economy (Resnick 2011). Urban slum dwellers describe high rates of crime, alcohol and drug abuse, and sexual violence. Government health clinics are overcrowded and lack basic medications, schools are understaffed, and sanitation and garbage collection are largely absent (FGDs, PLHIV groups, Ndola, June 11, 2014). Thus, despite Zambia's impressive growth rates, poverty and inequality are widespread. In 2014, 60 % of Zambians lived below the poverty line and the Gini coefficient was 0.56 (World Bank 2015b). In Malawi, these numbers were 50 % and 0.46 (World Bank 2015a). In 2012, 64 % of the population in Zambia and 67 % of the population in Malawi were living in multidimensional poverty, meaning that they experience multiple deprivations in education, health, and standard of living (UNDP 2013a, 5, 2013b, 5). Parts of Zambia and southern Malawi experience periodic food insecurity, with an annual "hunger season" from November to March (MVAC 2012; WFP 2015). High food prices contribute to this hunger, leading the World Food Programme (2014) to classify 22 % of Malawians and 48 % of Zambians as undernourished in 2012. A common concern among the PLHIV we interviewed was food insecurity, and statements like "How can I take ART on an empty stomach?" were not uncommon (see also Kalofonos 2010).

The countries have similar political experiences, with each adopting multiparty democracy in the early 1990s after protests by civil society groups (miners in Zambia; church leaders and students in Malawi) (see Bratton 1992; Newell 1995; Freston 2004). As of 2015, each country was rated "partly free" by Freedom House, because of limits on freedoms for the media and civil society, centralization of executive power, and high levels of corruption (Freedom House 2015a, b). Even though both countries have experienced two elections in which the ruling party lost (1991 and 2011 in Zambia; 1994 and 2014 in Malawi), opposition party leaders who came to power have done little to advance the countries' democratic prospects; alternative leadership is lacking (Simutanyi 2013; Chinsinga 2003).

The two countries share many common experiences with HIV and AIDS. As of 2013, data from sentinel surveys indicate that 13 % of Zambians aged 15–49 years old were HIV positive. Zambia's HIV rate has remained stubbornly high, and prevalence in urban areas is twice that in rural areas (18.2 % versus 9.1 %) (Zambia NAC 2014). In Malawi, prevalence in 2010 (the year of the most recent national survey) was 11 %. Prevalence was higher in the urban areas than rural areas (23 % versus 11 %) and in the Southern Region (14.5 %) as compared to the North (6.6 %) and the Center (7.6 %) (NSO and ICF Macro 2011, 196).

In both countries, women are disproportionately infected with HIV. In Zambia, 15 % of women aged 15–49 years were HIV positive in

2014, while 11 % of men were. Prevalence was highest among women aged 35–39 years old (24.2 % compared to 17.6 % for men in the same age group). By 2010, the gender gap in prevalence had widened in Malawi: prevalence for men had declined from 10 to 8 %, while it remained constant for women at 13 %. The largest disparity was in the 15–19 years age group (3.7 % among girls and 0.4 % among boys) and prevalence was highest among women aged 35–39 years (24 %) (NSO and ICF 2011, 196–197). Moreover, in both countries women dispro-portionately experience poverty and HIV (on Malawi see Anderson 2015, 61–95). They often take on much of the burden of care for HIV patients and AIDS orphans (Chimwaza and Watkins 2004), and they mitigate shortfalls in food production. Women act as "shock absorbers" in times of crisis, as their unpaid labor lessens the negative impact of neoliberal development (see Moser 1989).

The first AIDS cases emerged in the late 1980s in Malawi and Zambia, and both governments were slow to acknowledge the disease. Political commitment to AIDS only emerged after advocacy by civil society groups and increased funding from donors. Like most other African states, both set up national AIDS bodies (the National AIDS Council in Zambia and the National AIDS Commission in Malawi) with representatives from govern-ment, donor organizations, and civil society. Zambia has been praised for being one of the first African states to involve civil society organizations and faith-based health care providers in its AIDS response (Patterson 2011; Iliffe 2006). With Global Fund assistance, ART was made free in Malawi in 2004 and Zambia in 2005, and by 2013, 90 % of Zambians and 67 % of Malawians who needed AIDS treatment could access it (Global Fund 2013; Ntata 2007; GoM 2015, 38).

AIDS funding has led NGOs in both countries to concentrate on AIDS over other health issues. Additionally, AIDS monies have encouraged groups not usually involved with health issues to take up AIDS (Epstein 2007; Morfit 2011). The result has been a massive increase in the number of community initiatives to address AIDS, leading to what Whyte et al. (2013) have termed the "projectification of AIDS care." As PLHIV with access to ART live longer and regain their health, the disease has become normalized as a "part of life" and less of a concern for many Zambians and Malawians as compared to other issues. For example, Afrobarometer (2012, 41; 2013a, 49) found that 0 % of Zambians and Malawians thought AIDS was an important problem facing that country that govern-ment should address. In contrast, people in both countries emphasized unemployment, food security, crime and security, transportation, water, and health care services more broadly as crucial concerns.

The Research Design

This book is based on eight months of fieldwork conducted in Zambia (during 2007, 2009, 2011, and 2014) and eight months in Malawi (during 2005, 2006, 2007, 2011, and 2014). When we designed our research, our original goal was to examine advocacy among faith-based and secular PLHIV groups in Zambia and to investigate the gender dimensions of HIV in Malawi. Over time, we became interested in the nuances of agency that we observed within and alongside the formal research process. Our research question emerged from the ground: How are local actors in Zambia and Malawi simultaneously active within and dependent on donor structures?

What is particularly unique is that our multiyear span of research in two similar countries enables us to see changes in the AIDS enterprise and to assess the dynamism of local agency. The range of data from our multi-method approach allows us to examine the nuances of dependent agency from different angles. The data comes from NGO, government, and donor reports; interviews; local media sources; participant observations at clinics, trainings, and PLHIV group meetings; informal discussions; and focus group discussions (FGDs) with local affiliates of the Network of Zambian People Living with HIV and AIDS (NZP+), Zambian PLHIV groups linked to churches and clinics, and local affiliates of the National Association of People Living with HIV and AIDS in Malawi (NAPHAM). NZP+ and NAPHAM are national PLHIV organizations that were established early during the epidemic (NAPHAM in 1993 and NZP+ in 1996).

Key informant interviews were conducted with 152 donor and state officials, national and local NGO and FBO leaders, and AIDS activists in 2007 and 2011—80 in Zambia and 72 in Malawi. Interviewees were identified through the organizations that they represent, media stories, and recommendations from AIDS country experts, as well as through snowball sampling. Themes of interviews included government policies on AIDS, effectiveness of AIDS advocacy, relations with donors, changes over time in AIDS program priorities, and challenges in the AIDS response.

In 2011, we also held FGDs with support groups for PLHIV—57 in Zambia and 24 in Malawi. In Zambia, 33 groups were affiliated with

NZP+ and 24 with churches or AIDS clinics. Only four were located in a rural community; 26 were located in Lusaka; and 31 worked in Ndola, Kabwe, Kitwe, Mumbwa, and Chingola. Access to local groups was facilitated through church and clinic officials and NZP+ leaders, who invited participants, moderated sessions, and translated from English if needed. In Malawi, 22 groups were affiliated with NAPHAM, while the other two were accessed through local contacts. Half of the groups were in Karonga District in the north and the other half were in Zomba District in the south; groups were spread across urban, peri-urban, and rural districts. Access to Malawian groups was facilitated through the group's chairperson whom one of the authors met at a NAPHAM training and executive committee meeting.

Because gender was a focus in some of the Malawi research, two FGDs were conducted with almost all of the 24 Malawian support groups: one with men and one with women. The discussions were conducted in Chitumbuka in Karonga District and Chichewa in Zomba District, and a local research partner (a social worker with experience working in HIV and health) moderated the sessions while the researcher took notes. Most FGDs were embedded in regularly scheduled group meetings in both countries, giving research participants greater control over the norms and conduct of the session. All FGDs began by describing the project, asking for consent, answering questions about the research, and assuring participants that comments and organizational names would be kept anonymous. Themes for the FGDs included group activities, internal group dynamics, interactions with donors, group challenges, and motivations for belonging to the group. Discussions lasted roughly 90 minutes, were open to all members, and included up to 14 participants. Participants received no reward beyond snacks in most Zambian groups, while the groups in Malawi provided the research team with lunch as part of their regular meetings.

Zambian support groups had around 15 members. Most had been established around 2005, though three dated back to 2000. (Support groups founded before 2000 were rare, since many of their leaders and members had died without ART access.) Seven of the support groups in Zambia focused solely on caregiving, and these organizations had between 30 and 40 members, a number which included caregivers and PLHIV. (Caregivers sometimes were also HIV positive.) In Malawi, most of the support groups in Karonga had been established since 2008 and had between 15 and 50 members. The groups in Zomba formed in 2011, after the extension of NAPHAM to all districts and the establishment of the NAPHAM district office in 2011. Groups had between 30 and 100 members. In all of the groups, most members were women, reflecting the fact that HIV prevalence is higher among women than men in both countries (Zambia NAC 2014; GoM 2015); women are more likely than men to test for HIV, to access ART, and to participate in groups; and women have fewer opportunities for employment in the formal economy, a fact that may give them more flexible schedules for participating in PLHIV groups (Patterson 2015; Anderson 2015). Women's decision to join support groups may also illustrate their agency in societies where they are traditionally dependent on men; by joining the groups they choose to reveal their HIV status (despite family, marital, or societal stigma) in order to gain tangible and intangible benefits. (See Chapter 3 on gender and agency.) Despite women's participation, most groups in both countries tended to be led by men. The Malawian and Zambian groups resemble many other AIDS-related community organizations in Africa (see Burchardt 2013; Beckmann and Bujra 2010).

All of these groups did roughly the same tasks in both countries: they promoted ART adherence and HIV testing; they helped comembers with household chores and material needs; they provided psychosocial and spiritual support, health education, and care for orphans and vulnerable children; and, when donor funding was available, they engaged in income-generating projects like gardens, chicken-raising, or petty trade. These organizations also engaged in trainings and advocacy. In all groups, members spoke of their unity, as they faced common challenges of death, illness, suffering, discrimination, relationship difficulties surrounding HIV status, and poverty (FGDs, PLHIV groups, Lusaka, April 5, 2011; May 19, 2011; Zomba and Karonga, July–September 2011).

In addition, we conducted participant observations in 2011. In both countries, we observed support group meetings; the interactions that AIDS clinic officials, local group leaders, and PLHIV had with donors; and members' involvement in income-generation projects. One researcher observed HIV counselling processes and PLHIV experiences in two Zambian clinics (one was government affiliated and the other, church related). The other researcher participated in a week-long, national-level training workshop for representatives of support groups convened by the Malawi Network of People Living with HIV/AIDS (MANET+), an umbrella body for the networks of people living with HIV. This researcher also shadowed the work of the Zomba AIDS coordinator and attended two different week-long training workshops in Zomba District hosted by NAPHAM and the Malawi Network of AIDS Service Organisations (MANASO) and another one-day workshop in Karonga District convened by the District Interfaith AIDS Committee.

The participant observations of meetings, training sessions, and AIDS clinic activities enabled us to verify our interview and focus group data. They also allowed us to witness the discrepancies between the onstage public performances of interviews and FGDs and the offstage performances that may occur when subjects are engaged in other tasks like group meetings or projects. Observations also helped us to understand the meaning that those actors gave to their performances. Similar insights emerged from the informal discussions we had with individuals and groups as we got to know them over the course of the research. These conversations often occurred at unexpected moments: as we traveled to training sessions, waited for focus group members to arrive, and/or shared meals or refreshments.

It is important to recognize that the research process itself is also a site where power operates. We recognized the likelihood that actors would engage in performances of compliance and extraversion within those power structures. The semi-structured format of interviews was intended to give the respondents more control, and we stressed that there were no right or wrong answers to the questions we posed. When we visited the support groups for PLHIV, we, as well as our informants, emphasized that we were not donor officials, and thus, had no resources to share; we also explained that our goal was not to assess particular groups for funders. In the case of the key informant interviews in particular, the respondents were in a position to represent the organizations they work for and this fact engendered a preoccupation in performing their professional knowledge and expertise (Interviews and FGDs, Lusaka, Ndola, Livingstone, Kabwe, Lilongwe, Zomba, and Karonga, April—September 2011). As these representatives continually repeated the "accepted" rhetoric it became normalized in their own understandings; as Scott (1990, 9–10) explains, the performer's face grows to fit the mask of the performance. On a number of occasions these understandings infiltrated the speech of respondents when they met the authors outside of the formal interviews (Informal discussions, NGO representatives, Lilongwe, Lusaka, Ndola, Zomba, and Karonga, April-September 2011). It is important to recognize that it is problematic to determine whether or not a performance is genuine (Scott 1990, 4), with every performance subject to a degree of interpretation by the researchers and the actors themselves. Yet we were less concerned about the genuineness of sentiments expressed than about the fact that these performances were repeatedly given and that they construct a reality that observers and performers alike may come to believe.

NEXT STEPS

This chapter has focused on dependent agency, or the agency that individuals living in conditions of aid dependency may utilize. We have highlighted how donor competition, foreign aid uncertainty, and development theories that urge local participation may provide opportunities for agency. We have also alluded to strategies that dependent actors might use, including performances of compliance, extraversion, and resistance below the line. How do local actors respond to HIV exceptionalism and the myriad of opportunities and constraints that accompany it?

The rest of the book tackles this question. Chapter 2 interrogates the conditions for dependent agency in the context of Malawi and Zambia during 2011, a time when AIDS funding had retracted, donors had started to replace food support for PLHIV with income-generating projects, both governments were embroiled in corruption scandals around AIDS money, and the large number of AIDS groups that had formed in the mid-2000s increasingly competed for resources. We explore how this environment led to particular conditions under which dependent agency was possible. Chapter 3 then tackles the strategies of dependent agency. We begin by acknowledging that local agents have multiple and overlapping objectives, such as building community, helping their kin, gaining local influence, and accessing material resources. Crucially, we show that strategies of dependent agents can change over time. For example, Zambian church-related groups have used Christian language both in performances of compliance and in extraversion. Many groups have engaged in extraversion, though the ways they have done so have changed with time. In Chapter 4, we highlight the effects of strategies of dependent agents, particularly for PLHIV solidarity and for donors' actions. In the process, we point to why these lessons matter as donors seek to promote sustainable development. We assert that lessons related to AIDS are applicable to other areas of health and development.

We conclude by questioning the ramifications of dependent agency for democratic citizenship and socioeconomic development in Africa.

NOTE

1. We use the acronym PLHIV to stand for both the single and plural form, or *person or people living with HIV*.

CHAPTER 2

Unique Opportunities in a Dynamic Aid Architecture: The Conditions for Agency

Abstract Dynamic donor programs create conditions for dependent agency. Increases in AIDS funding in the mid-2000s led to new community-level programs and structures. The 2008–2009 global recession, deteriorating donor–recipient relations, and corruption scandals then caused a slowdown of AIDS monies after 2009. Donors' priorities shifted from a rapidly scaled-up emergency response to sustaining that response. The dynamic aid architecture provided "wiggle room" for dependent agents, as local people living with HIV responded to the new issues and opportunities that emerged in the AIDS enterprise.

Keywords Donor programs · Conditions for dependent agency · Aid dependency · Donor–recipient relations · Malawi · Zambia

In 2009, several bilateral donors withheld funding to the Zambian Ministry of Health (MoH), after charges of corruption. The following year a Global Fund audit revealed corruption in the management of its grants to Malawi (OIG 2012, 1). By 2011, the Global Fund had suspended grants to several Zambian recipients and withdrawn from the HIV pooled-funding mechanism in Malawi because of alleged fraud and misappropriation. In Malawi, the Global Fund then rejected new proposals for funding, and in both countries, other donors suspended money for AIDS. While these donor actions were more significant in Malawi, in both

© The Author(s) 2017
E.-L. Anderson, A.S. Patterson, *Dependent Agency in the Global Health Regime*, DOI 10.1057/978-1-137-58148-8_2

countries they negatively affected AIDS programs, particularly as they came on the heels of the 2008–2009 global recession. These funding decreases followed several years of expansion in donor AIDS spending and programs. Backed into a funding corner, our dependent agents seem like victims of entrenched corruption that negatively affects service delivery and is symptomatic of deeper processes of neopatrimonial governance, as well as vacillating foreign aid priorities which may ignore poor people's needs (Afrobarometer 2013b; Englebert and Dunn 2013). One Zambian PLHIV blogged, "[The] Global Fund drought [is] a recipe for higher HIV incidence," and another PLHIV blamed donor cuts for 14 deaths from tuberculosis (Syed 2011; *IRIN News*, March 14, 2011). Similarly, *Médecins sans Frontières* (MSF 2011) said that the rejection of Malawi's Global Fund grant proposal would threaten the continuity of antiretroviral (ARV) programs for those already enrolled and undermine commitment to the WHO's new ART directives. Yet, as this chapter and Chapter 3 argue, even these dependent contexts provide opportunities for agents to act, react, speak, remain silent, and/or reframe their options. Situated within specific social sites (Scott 1990, 14), dependent agents may manoeuver around constraints, using social and cultural resources and even donors' own objectives and rhetoric to achieve their goals. This is particularly the case where aid structures changed, creating new spaces for agentic activities.

In Chapter 1, we highlighted the broader economic, political, and social context of our two country case studies. In this chapter, we drill down to the specific aspects of AIDS programming and donor funding in order to understand how the context in Malawi and Zambia at the time of this study presented unique opportunities for agency. Our goal is to highlight what we referred to in Chapter 1 as the "conditions" for agency. (The next chapter tackles the "strategies" that agents use.) These conditions include the multitude of dynamic donor programs which reflect donors' heterogeneous and shifting preferences; donors' own rhetoric, espoused norms, and ideologies; Western views of Africa as poverty-stricken and weak; and donors' own dependence on local actors to achieve their objectives. Because we collected data over several years, we are able to analyze these conditions during a period when AIDS funding surged and AIDS was treated as an emergency (the mid-2000s) and a period when donors cut funding and pressed for project sustainability (post-2009).

In this chapter we detail the changes in the AIDS enterprise from the mid-2000s until 2014. We first demonstrate how the "ramping up" of

AIDS funding in the mid-2000s created new programs and structures at the community level. We then show how the 2008–2009 global recession, deteriorating donor–recipient relations, and corruption scandals led to the "slowing down" of AIDS money after 2009. In Zambia, funding leveled off and some community AIDS groups lost resources, while in Malawi, donors drastically cut AIDS funds. In both countries, donors changed their priorities from rapid scale up in an emergency to sustaining the AIDS response. Though many donor-constructed AIDS institutions continued after adoption of the sustainability model, competition for resources in communities became more apparent. Changes in donor priorities created opportunities for dependent agents to utilize the strategies we analyze in Chapter 3.

THE "RAMPING UP" OF AIDS FUNDING: GLOBAL ATTENTION, LOCAL MOBILIZATION

By the mid-2000s, the AIDS crisis in Zambia and Malawi had received great attention from donors. Hundreds of international NGOs and FBOs worked in each country, often partnering with local community groups or churches (Kelly and Birdsall 2010, 1582). In 2003, Zambia was chosen as one of the 15 focus countries in the PEPFAR program, and between 2004 and 2008, it received around USD 800 million from PEPFAR (SIECUS 2008). Zambia also received USD 635 million between 2003 and 2015 from the Global Fund for its AIDS programs, and another USD 24 million for its TB/HIV efforts. These funds have come through over 20 grants for HIV/AIDS, HIV/tuberculosis, malaria, and tuberculosis (Global Fund 2015c).

Malawi was not an original PEPFAR focus country, though it has received between USD 20 million and 95 million annually from the program since 2006 (PEPFAR 2016). For Malawi, the Global Fund has been the major donor. In 2002, the country secured USD 196 million to support its integrated national response through the National Strategic Framework with a main focus on care and support, particularly in the provision of ART to 25,000 people over 5 years. This led to a national-level policy impetus focusing on the prevention of mother-to-child transmission (PMTCT) and the provision of ART (Kemp et al. 2003, 16). The Global Fund was the major donor to the National AIDS Commission (NAC) in Malawi and provided two-thirds of the funds between 2003 and

2010 for the National HIV and AIDS Action Framework (equating to a total of USD 248.3 million) (Malawi NAC Financial Monitoring Reports, 30 June 2010 cited in OIG 2012, 35–36). By 2010, when the aforementioned Global Fund audit occurred, Malawi had received seven grants totaling USD 460 million (OIG 2012, 1). In both countries, the EU and other bilateral donors also increased foreign assistance for health. For example, Sweden, Zambia's largest health sector donor, pledged a total of USD 153 million over the 2006–2010 period (*Lancet*, August 8, 2015). The United Kingdom, Malawi's largest bilateral health donor, increased its support to health from USD 31 million in 2003–2004 to USD 58 million in 2007–2008 (NAO 2009, 18).

On the one hand, donors' generosity in both Zambia and Malawi seemed to be a continuation of increased partnership that emerged after the countries' transitions to democracy in the early 1990s and their moves to embrace market economies. In Zambia this was particularly the case under the late president Frederick Chiluba (Szeftel 2000), while Malawi had long been considered a "strong liberaliser" (Peiffer and Englebert 2012, 358). Donors also rewarded efforts to fight corruption in both countries: for example, in 2005 they reduced Zambia's USD 7.2 billion external debt to USD 500 million (*IRIN News*, May 27, 2009; Taylor 2006), and the US government pledged a 50 % increase in developmental assistance of USD 5 billion annually to Malawi through the US Millennium Challenge Account (*IRIN News*, May 12 2005).

On the other hand, donors' objectives in the AIDS fight seemed more complicated than just historic relations. First, they seemed to funnel AIDS money to both countries because of international mobilization and local actions, many of which echoed donors' desire to support civil society (Harbeson et al. 1994). In the early 2000s, the Zambian AIDS orphan crisis received high levels of publicity through the awareness-raising campaigns of the Global AIDS Alliance and the international FBO World Vision (Hunter and Williamson 1997; Interview, World Vision official, Washington, DC, April 14, 2005). Former Zambian President Kenneth Kaunda demonstrated political commitment to AIDS (a value donors found essential in the AIDS response; see UN 2001, 15) when he publicly acknowledged that his son had died of AIDS (*New York Times*, October 5, 1987). Similarly, the former Malawian president Bakili Muluzi announced at the launch of the country's first HIV/AIDS policy in 2004 that his brother had died of AIDS 3 years previously (*BBC*, February 10, 2004).

Zambian and Malawian civil society organizations had played a crucial role in reestablishing democracy in the 1990s (Bratton 1999; Bartlett 2000; Newell 1995), and donors praised their continued activism on the AIDS issue. (Civil society has played a larger role in the AIDS response than originally acknowledged. See Rau 2006, 294.) For example, Bishop Joshua Banda of the Northmead Assemblies of God, a Pentecostal mega-church in Lusaka, and several Catholic leaders in Ndola developed AIDS care and support programs (Patterson 2013; Interview, FBO official, August 16, 2007). Similarly, the Roman Catholic, Assemblies of God, and Seventh Day Adventist churches in Malawi developed relief, development, and HBC departments that assisted PLHIV (Interviews, FBO officials, Limbe and Lilongwe, July 12–24, 2007). International donors praised civil society, with a technical advisor at the Canadian International Development Agency (CIDA) highlighting its continuing importance in the AIDS response, despite some division between the churches (Interview, Lilongwe, July 26, 2007). These civil society actors also had representation in AIDS policymaking in Zambia, with the Churches Health Association of Zambia (CHAZ) and the Zambia National AIDS Network (ZNAN) sitting on the National AIDS Council (NAC) and the Country Coordinating Mechanism (Interview, donor official, Lusaka, August 12, 2007). Zambia's first Global Fund application included four principal recipients, two of which were ZNAN and CHAZ. (Principal recipients submit grant proposals and if successful, manage grant monies, often providing funds to subrecipients.) As a symbol of donors' appreciation for Zambian civil society involvement in the AIDS response, the UN Secretary General appointed Elizabeth Mataka, the chairperson of ZNAN, to serve as UN Special Envoy on HIV/AIDS to Africa in 2007 (*Lancet*, December 1, 2007).

Donors also supported the countries' AIDS efforts because of norms related to AIDS treatment (see Chapter 1) and because of the perception that Africa needs the West. Calling for treatment in Africa as he announced the formation of the PEPFAR program, for example, US President George W. Bush (2003) said, "In an age of miraculous medicines, no person should have to hear [the words] 'We have no medicines...Go home and die'." The notion of Western obligation to help Africans which is embedded in this statement opened the door for new AIDS programs. As Chapter 3 indicates, dependent agents could capitalize on these norms and perceptions of "needy" Africa in the agentic strategies of extraversion and performances of compliance.

While donors supported the AIDS response because of their past involvement in these two countries, global norms, views on African dependence, and the two countries' own efforts, it is important to recognize that donors also depended on the recipient countries in order to meet their own AIDS program objectives. PEPFAR, for example, set global goals for 2003–2008 of treating two million people with ART, preventing seven million new HIV infections, and providing support and care to ten million people who were infected with or affected by AIDS. As mandated in legislation, these goals drove the selection of countries for the PEPFAR program; countries needed to have a sizeable number of HIV-positive people, a fact that meant countries with small populations which still had high HIV rates (e.g., Swaziland) did not become focus countries. With its roughly 100,000 PLHIV, Zambia's inclusion helped the program show results (Patterson 2006). Additionally, the dozens of international NGOs and FBOs that worked in both countries needed community groups and PLHIV in order to meet goals. In Malawi, Action Aid, for example, partnered with the Coalition of Women Living with HIV and AIDS (COWLHA) to meet its strategic priority of fostering women's rights. In 2007, when one author interviewed Action Aid's Gender Network National Coordinator, the respondent invited the Head of COWLHA to the meeting as a means of demonstrating Action Aid's work on gender and HIV/AIDS (Interview, Lilongwe, July 17, 2007). One interviewee at a US church that gave financial support to a Zambian FBO explained that his church members "depended" on the Zambian FBO so they could "fulfil the Gospel's call for Christians to care for the sick, homeless, orphans, and widows" (Interview, FBO partner, Chicago, IL, August 30, 2013). In short, the well-being of the American parishioners' spiritual life partially rested on the relationship with a Zambian FBO. The dependence of donors on Zambians and Malawians could create the opportunity for local agency.

It was apparent that donors appreciated both countries' AIDS activities. In interviews in 2007, donors praised Zambia's AIDS efforts, which included the provision of free ART access after 2005, the removal of user fees at clinics in 2006, the establishment of the NAC, the development of a multisectoral National Strategic Framework, and the incorporation of civil society into the country's AIDS response (Interview, Zambia NAC official, Lusaka, August 14, 2007). Donors praised the fact that these policies were made through a highly consultative process that included donors, government, and civil society (Interview, bilateral donor, Lusaka, August 13, 2007). Donors and

NGO officials asserted that the country was on the right track: "The NAC is finally getting somewhere," "Government is paying attention to the problem" (Interviews, International NGO official and DfID official, Lusaka, August 15, 2007). Even when respondents criticized AIDS efforts—"The government has minimal commitment" or "Decision-making in the NAC has not adequately included the voices of people with the disease"—they also urged patience as the country developed new health structures (Interviews, CHAZ official and DfID official, Lusaka, August 15–16, 2007). They said it would take time to develop an efficient, effective response because of the magnitude of the crisis and because of Zambia's low health care capacity (Interview, International NGO official, Lusaka, August 15, 2007).

In Malawi, DfID praised NAC for its "highly effective" leadership, the "significant progress" it had made, and for "increasing donor confidence" (DfID 2012a, 5–6). The establishment of NAC in 2001 and the Department of Nutrition, HIV, and AIDS in the Office of the President and Cabinet (to whom NAC reports) in 2004 was a widely highlighted move toward a more centralized and coordinated response that would enhance government leadership (Interviews, DfID official, CIDA specialist, CIDA technical advisor, and World Bank official, Lilongwe, July 26–27, 2007). NAC oversaw the disbursal of funding and until 2012, provided grants to more than 1000 public and civil society organizations (DfID Malawi 2012a, 5–6). To increase collaboration between donors and government, a health sector-wide approach (SWAp) evolved to replace the fragmented vertical disease-based approach (Pearson 2010, 7). From 2004 until June 2010, the key pool donors of DfID (USD 120 million), Government of Norway (USD 104 million), the Global Fund (USD 57 million), and the World Bank (USD 10 million) supported the National HIV and AIDS Action Framework (MoH Financial Monitoring Reports, June 30, 2010 cited in OIG 2012, 11). And other discrete donors aligned their support to the national priorities and participated in the HIV and AIDS Development Group to harmonize, align, and coordinate their efforts.

This is not to say that these efforts to support the Malawian response were not without challenges. As one respondent explained in 2007, NAC had not yet been supported by an act of parliament, and it did not have the mandate to request the data it required to coordinate the response, especially from organizations that did not receive NAC funding (Interview, CIDA technical advisor, Lilongwe, July 26, 2007). Also, sometimes donors acted in ways that were at odds with the pooled-funding mechanism, such as when Canada withdrew its support in 2007–2008 because of political changes and Sweden withdrew support in 2009 (DfID Malawi 2012a, 7). Despite these challenges, there was relatively high donor support and optimism in Malawi until 2010. At the individual and community level, donor funding enabled many PLHIV to access ART. By 2011 in Malawi, 67 % of people who needed AIDS medications had ART access and the number of registered clients increased from 10,000 in 2004 to 277,000; most of these PLHIV received free treatment (Ministry of Health, Malawi ART Programme Quarterly Report, June 2011 cited in DfID Malawi 2012a, 4). By 2012 in Zambia, 82 % of people who needed treatment had access to ART and mortality from AIDS had declined over 50 % (see Global Fund 2014). Donor monies paid for care and support programs for PLHIV, as well as AIDS orphans and their caregivers. By 2011, PEPFAR had provided ART in Zambia to over 350,000 PLHIV and care and support to over 900,000 individuals (PEPFAR 2011). In order to facilitate these programs, new community organizations developed. These organizations sought to promote HIV testing and ART adherence, with the latter being a crucial concern for donors. Because of their large role in Global Fund grants in Zambia, CHAZ and ZNAN took on a leadership role in supporting community organizational development, working through church partners (for CHAZ) and community-based organizations (for ZNAN). Additionally, because PEPFAR provided substantial funding through international NGOs and FBOs from its inception in 2003 until 2006 (Patterson 2006), these nonstate actors often collaborated with local-level partners.

This structure of multiple national and international NGOs and FBOs that implemented programs had several implications, all of which created opportunities for agency. First, many of the implementing groups were outside of the government's control. This fact enabled the government to claim credit for nonstate actors' successes, such as when CHAZ quickly increased the number of PLHIV on treatment (Interview, DfID official, Lusaka, August 15, 2007). In the process, government "looked good" to its citizens, though it was not directly responsible for funding or implementing half of Zambia's ART programs (see Fox 2014). But CHAZ and ZNAN could also be viewed as competitors with government, a fact that could benefit these groups as they worked with donor states like the United States that have tended to be suspicious of government ministries (Interviews, DfID official and ZNAN official, Lusaka, August 15 and August 20, 2007; on undermining state ministries, see Harman 2009).

Second, the resulting AIDS structures resembled what Susan Whyte et al. (2013, 140) term a "projectified" environment, where the "landscape of health care blossomed with an array of programs instead of just one standard package of care provided through the existing government health care system." In Zambia and Malawi, neighborhoods, churches, and clinics developed their own programs that recruited PLHIV and monitored their medications and health. Support groups for PLHIV proliferated. In one Lusaka slum neighborhood, for example, at least eight different groups existed, each with 15–20 members. The condition of multiple donors tied to a plethora of local partners created an opening for agentic individuals: it was not uncommon during the fieldwork in Zambia to encounter some of the same people at multiple support group meetings. Support groups complained that people "skipped around from group to group," looking for better benefits such as food parcels, links to clinics with possible employment, and funds for orphan care (Interview, NZP+ leader, Lusaka, March 21, 2011). This "shifting between groups" made it difficult to inculcate a sense of "belonging" among some group members (FGD, PLHIV group, Lusaka, March 22, 2011).

Third, because there was a multitude of donors competing at the local level with different emphases in their community AIDS work (e.g., orphan care, care for PLHIV, educating about HIV prevention, and support for PLHIV), donors' numerous local partners could define and redefine themselves, as they played to the particular concerns of specific donors. The division of labor among donors was mirrored in local community groups: for example, churches often focused on HBC while community groups worked on ART adherence and HIV education and testing. This division of labor also meant that organizations that had not previously been involved in local health and development initiatives could "get into the AIDS game" to gain access to resources (Interview, AIDS policy expert, Washington, DC, April 15, 2005). For example, churches, some of which had never engaged in social service delivery, now developed HBC projects (FGD, PLHIV group, Lusaka, March 10, 2011; Interviews, FBO officials, Limbe and Lilongwe, July 12–24, 2007). These initiatives were possible because of the large number of donors, many with their own special requirements for AIDS programs.

As Chapter 3 further illustrates, a final outcome was that donors became increasingly concerned about working with "authentic" groups in local communities. The rise of the "briefcase NGOs" had donors worried, particularly as stories about such groups emerged in the media with the rise of AIDS funding (*Guardian*, May 2, 2014; Edwards and Hulme 1996). Authentic groups were those with deep roots in the community; they had not simply been formed when donors arrived and wanted to start a project. Authentic groups were tied to respected local leaders (such as pastors or imams) who knew the community's inhabitants and their needs; they also had "permanent" structures (such as church buildings) in many communities, and they reflected community values, reciprocal ties among members, and the moral economy of dependence (Marshall and van Saanen 2007). Being "authentic" could open the door for donor support.

As donors began to work with communities, their goal was to test as many people as possible for HIV in order to get them enrolled in ART treatment. Donors depended on rapid scale up to meet their goals and to illustrate to key constituencies that they were acting on AIDS (Benton 2015). Prior to the scale up in ART, many people did not test for the HIV virus until they were very ill; people perceived that it was useless to know their HIV status because infection meant certain death (MSF 2001) Some also avoided testing, because they assumed HIV was highly transmissible and therefore, they would test positive (Kaler and Watkins 2010). Many focus group participants in Zambia mentioned that knowing that one was HIV positive but being unable to do anything about it would be tortuous (FGDs, PLHIV groups, Lusaka, March 2 and March 9, 2011). ART access has changed this dynamic, with HIV testing increasing in Zambia by 50 % (Wilson 2016). To urge testing, donors gave food supplements to people who were HIV positive, and they urged PLHIV to join support groups and to disclose their status. One informant said that food supplements were an "entry point," or a way of "bringing more people who are hiding out into the open." The informant continued: "We were just buying people...because food is how we could attract a poor person" (FGD, NZP+ leader, Mumbwa, April 15, 2011). In addition to urging testing, food helped PLHIV who were sick and thus, unable to work, to adhere to ART, and for donors, adherence was crucial to prevent ARV resistance (Interviews, donor official, Lusaka, February 23, 2011; NAC official, Lusaka, August 14, 2007). In short, donors depended on local groups and food distribution to ensure adherence so that their programs could be deemed effective.

Food distribution facilitated HIV testing and although this tended to occur primarily for women who were tested at antenatal clinics, in Malawi "couple testing" initiatives provided food support to couples who attended the clinics to test together (Interview, WFP official, Lilongwe, July 23, 2007). And yet, even with food distribution, men often shunned testing, fearing that if they were HIV positive, the disease would prevent them from working and providing for their families, and it would undermine their masculinity (Skovdal et al. 2011). One clinic counsellor in Lusaka said, "The men will be dying, and have to be brought in by neighbors or family in a wheelbarrow before they will test" (Interview, Lusaka, March 2, 2011).

Food distribution led to the formation of hundreds of the aforementioned support groups, since it was through these groups that food parcels were distributed. These groups were intended to increase PLHIV's adherence to ART, to help them "live positively" by providing education on good nutrition and safer sex, and to encourage them to act as spokespeople for HIV prevention (Rasmussen 2013). Modeled on Western AIDS activists' mobilization in the 1980s, these groups were rooted in the assumption that HIV education would enable PLHIV to live, work, and love despite their status and that disclosure of one's HIV status was crucial for living this healthy, positive life. Formation of groups also related to the idea that PLHIV would become activists who demanded human rights protection, AIDS programs, and treatment (Robins 2004; Heywood 2009). While several scholars have disputed these assumptions (Nguyen 2010; Patterson 2015; Rasmussen 2013; Anderson 2015; Beckmann and Bujra 2010; Benton 2015), we are interested in the ways that these assumptions created opportunities for PLHIV agency. As the next chapter illustrates, when PLHIV's actions and rhetoric—or their performances of compliance—aligned with donors' assumptions, they could gain attention, support, and local influence.

Food programs legitimated selective benefits for some in society, because donors had implicitly created new definitions of who "deserved" help (Siplon 2013; Nguyen 2010, 177, 186; Benton 2015). Hungry PLHIV were distinguished from hungry people who were HIV negative, with the latter being ineligible for food. Yet in 2006, the cost of basic foodstuffs per month in Lusaka's slums was twice the average monthly household income and the vast majority of slum residents did not eat three meals a day (Resnick 2011, 148). Donors' food distribution programs benefited PLHIV, but many HIV-negative people needed the benefits that PLHIV-exclusive projects provided (FGD, caregiver group, Ndola, May 21, 2011). Donors' focus on PLHIV for benefits provided an opportunity to "remake oneself," or to redefine one's identity to fit into this donor-determined context. Chapter 3 further highlights how local PLHIV used the strategy of extraversion to high-light their HIV status to meet donors' goal of working with HIV-positive individuals. Chapter 4 then analyzes how the use of HIV status as a tool to gain resources can undermine solidarity among all poor Malawians and Zambians.

Devised and funded in the West but implemented by local organizations, donor programs created opportunities for individuals who understood local dynamics and donor priorities to serve as brokers. These brokers were necessary in a hierarchical AIDS enterprise with many actors who often did not directly interact with one another; the hierarchy created spaces for innovation and translation (Patterson 2016). For example, the Global Fund provided grants to CHAZ, which then worked with local churches and ecumenical councils. CHAZ officials and local pastors acted as brokers. PEPFAR funded international FBOs and NGOs, which partnered with community groups such as NZP+. Zambian staff at these donor agencies, as well as community leaders like NZP+ district coordinators, translated between each level. Being a broker required a delicate dance between donors and local constituencies, each of which had expectations for the broker. One CHAZ official explained how hard it was to walk this tightrope in regards to its Global Fund grants. He said that many churches thought they would be able to access money after CHAZ got its first Global Fund grant, but the reality was that many churches lacked the capacity to submit competitive proposals or manage projects. ("They just did not realize what it takes to run a project.") When CHAZ officials tried to explain, some local church leaders became irate, leading to tensions between CHAZ and church denomina-tions (Interview, CHAZ official, Lusaka, April 16, 2009). A similar situation emerged with ZNAN, when PLHIV groups felt excluded from its funding decisions (*Lancet*, December 1, 2007). Despite these pressures, being a broker provided opportunities for recognition, invitations to trainings, pos-sible employment, and resources. As Chapter 3 shows, these benefits were particularly available if brokers adopted donors' rhetoric and ideals in per-formances of compliance.

In summary, the increase in donor resources for AIDS, and the devel-opment of a plethora of local AIDS organizations, created opportunities for local agency. Some opportunities emerged from donors' multiple pre-ferences, their concerns about authenticity, their views of "deservedness," their need for brokers, and their own dependence on local partners to achieve results. These factors made agency possible.

SLOWING DOWN OR LEVELING OFF AIDS FUNDING: FINANCIAL CRISIS AND CORRUPTION

When we returned to Zambia and Malawi in 2011 for more research, donors had become more circumspect about their AIDS efforts. The global financial crisis and corruption charges that undermined donors' trust led to this change. Even in this context of limited resources and donor suspicion, though, dependent agency was possible. In fact, as the next chapter indicates, cuts in funding made extraversion more powerful and the need to perfect performances of compliance, more essential.

The global financial crisis caused a contraction of the economies of the donor countries, with implications for their foreign assistance programs (GoM 2011, 10). While both countries depend heavily on foreign aid for the AIDS response, the global crisis had different effects on each. For Zambia, both project and budgetary aid did not decline in the aggregate; the economic crisis was short-lived and mostly affected trade and foreign investments. By 2010, Zambia had returned to precrisis growth levels (Ndulo et al. 2010, 13). In contrast, Malawi's economic situation was particularly negative (see DfID Malawi 2012b, 2), and the effects lingered in that country until at least 2014. (We acknowledge that both countries' economies were hurt by the decline in China's economic growth in 2015–2016, and for Zambia, the fall of commodity prices. See *New York Times*, January 26, 2016).

While the two countries were unevenly affected by the 2008–2009 global recession, both were impacted by donors' concerns about corruption in AIDS funding. Here again, though, Malawi was more negatively impacted than Zambia was. In Zambia, the governments of Sweden and the Netherlands reported in 2009 that they had suspended USD 33 million in aid to the MoH over the embezzlement of USD 2 million. Several other donors followed, leading to a freeze in the pooled funding for the MoH as well as cuts in other projects such as road construction (*IRIN News*, May 27, 2009; *Lusaka Times*, June 16, 2010). Then in late 2010, the Global Fund announced that three of Zambia's four principal recipients had mismanaged funds: the MoH had misused or misreported USD 14 million; the Ministry of Finance and National Planning, USD 1.5 million; and ZNAN, USD 1.8 million. The Global Fund demanded that all three repay monies and that the UN Development Programme (UNDP) replace the MoH as a principal recipient. While the government sought to repay some of the funds that the ministry had mismanaged, it distanced itself from ZNAN, even though some AIDS activists called for government support. The scandal had particularly negative effects on ZNAN and, more broadly, its CBO partners, especially after ZNAN was alleged to have purchased expensive cars and furniture for staff members' personal use, paid staff members exorbitant salaries, and had given grants to some politically connected (and potentially fraudulent) groups such as the Maureen Mwanawasa Community Initiative (led by Zambia's former first lady) (*IRIN News*, March 14, 2011; Global Fund 2010). CHAZ was relatively untarnished in the scandal, heightening donors' overall positive views of the FBO (Interviews, DfID official, Lusaka, August 15, 2007; International donor, Lusaka, February 23, 2011). While UNDP moved relatively rapidly to take over the MoH grants, ZNAN's grants were frozen for over a year until CHAZ took over their management. ZNAN was disbanded in late 2011 (Garmaise 2011).

As a result, funding to health care providers in Zambia decreased 40 %, programs in maternal and new born health, malaria, and respiratory infections suffered, and antenatal coverage dropped from 95 % in early 2009 to 78 % in 2010 (*Lancet*, August 8, 2015). PLHIV's health suffered: many clinics experienced ART shortages during 2011. Stock outs increased the economic burden for PLHIV, who had to incur greater transportation costs to visit clinics more frequently in order to get their medications. The funding cuts also negatively impacted some community groups. NZP+, a subrecipient of ZNAN-administered grants, was no longer able to pay its district coordinators a stipend, a fact that hampered morale; NZP+ also limited some of its advocacy efforts such as Global AIDS Day events and HIV testing campaigns (FGD, PLHIV group, Lusaka, March 30, 2011; Interview, PLHIV, Lusaka, March 21, 2011). These were real costs for donors' withdrawal. Unlike in the Malawi case, by 2011 donors seemed willing to continue funding Zambia's AIDS efforts, though with some stipulations on how funds for community groups could be used (e.g., local coordinators could not receive salaries). Throughout the Global Fund scandal, PEPFAR never cut its funding, and in 2012, Zambia received another Global Fund grant for USD 102 million for ARVs and in 2014, it signed a grant of USD 245 million for ARVs and TB/HIV prevention and treatment (Ravelo 2012; Global Fund 2015d).

Until 2010 it seemed that Malawi was performing well in terms of accountability for donor funds. There had been a Memorandum of Understanding (MOU) in place between the NAC (the principal recipient for Global Fund money) and the Anti-Corruption Bureau since 2008, and this was renewed in 2010 until 2013. The Secretary for Nutrition, HIV, and AIDS in the Office of President and Cabinet, Mary Shawa, announced that the renewal of the MOU would further help to instill trust in donors: "Malawi has a good reputation to donors [sic]. Global Fund is no longer giving money to some countries which were the first recipients, but Malawi has maintained the good record all along, which is a milestone" (*Africa News*, November 27, 2010).

Despite this positive portrayal, in February 2010 the Global Fund Board rejected a proposal for USD 4 million for an application to adopt new WHO treatment directives, reportedly due to failures to address the restructuring of the Central Medical Stores (the government's medicines purchasing and dispersal agency) and other critical issues (*Africa Review*, December 31, 2010). A Global Fund audit in 2010 revealed a lack of accountability and transparency in terms of fiscal management of grants (OIG 2012, 1–2). In December 2010, a proposal to the Global Fund for USD 560 million to support its national HIV/AIDS response for a 5-year period was denied with no option of resubmission, reportedly because of the country's laws criminalizing homosexuality and prostitution (*Africa Review*, December 31, 2010). Furthermore, deteriorating donor relations exacerbated the retraction of external funds. In April 2011, the British High Commissioner to Malawi, Fergus Cochrane-Dyet, was expelled for accusing then President Bingu wa Mutharika of being autocratic in a leaked cable (*BBC*, April 27, 2011). And then in July 2012, DfID suspended its budgetary support due to concerns over economic management, governance, and human rights (DfID Malawi 2012b, 2). Similarly, Germany withheld part of its aid for alleged human rights violations by the government (*IPS*, June 9, 2011).

After its 2010 audit, the Global Fund opted out of SWAp pooled funding in August 2011 and became a discrete donor; it also chose to use alternative supply systems instead of the Central Medical Stores to purchase pharmaceuticals and other health products (OIG 2012, 53). This followed on the heels of Global Fund concerns in 2009 about SWAp funding because "it did not comply with the minimum conditions in terms of assessment of performance, involvement of the Global Fund in the governance mechanisms, reports against budgeted program areas, account for each donor's annual contributions and performance-based funding" (OIG 2012, 10). The Global Fund also suspended its Round 11 grant to Malawi in 2012 (DfID Malawi 2012a, 6), and it required the Malawian government to refund USD 4 million over a 2-year period because of spending that was ineligible or not adequately supported with documents (OIG 2012, 1–2). This retraction had a knock-on effect and the other donors such as DfID followed (Interview, donor technical advisor, Lilongwe, July 26, 2014). As a result, in 2012, the NAC only received 60 % of its USD 132 million budget with a funding gap of USD 58 million (DfID Malawi 2012a, 7).

The lack of resources in Malawi led to a funding crisis in the health sector, particularly in national HIV programs (Interview, donor HIV expert, Lilongwe, July 26, 2014). The retraction of Global Fund support in particular had a considerable impact because the national program relies heavily on those resources for the procurement of ARVs, HIV test kits, and related drugs, items which none of the other pooled-funding partners purchase (DfID Malawi 2012a, 5–6). Here Malawi contrasted with Zambia, since the majority of ARVs in Zambia were purchased through PEPFAR (Zambia NAC 2014). *Médecins sans Frontières* warned that funding cuts threatened the treatment for patients already on ART and that the country would not be able to meet the WHO's new ART guidelines to change first-line treatment, introduce earlier treatment, and improve PMTCT programs (MSF 2011). During the 2011 fieldwork, the negative effects of funding cuts for local AIDS projects and the communities where they operated were apparent. The city and district AIDS coordinators for NAPHAM and other local NGOs highlighted their lack of resources and delays in the release of funds (Interviews, AIDS coordinators and NGO representatives, Zomba and Karonga, June—July 2011). One HIV/AIDS coordinator at an NGO explained how his organization was struggling in the country's shifting funding situation:

We have tried our best because of the problems with funding that we are having. We have had a lot of donors: NAC, we have USAID now, we had DFID, CIDA, and JICA, now DFID pulled out, NAC is pulling out (at the end of June the funding expires), now we just have this donor only, USAID . . . 110 people are losing their jobs as a result of the NAC pull out. People doing HIV have to leave countrywide because they are cutting the HIV testing and counselling and outreach programs. . . . Maybe tomorrow funding will come. Today no funding. Maybe tomorrow condoms, tomorrow not condoms. No test kits, next time test kits. So people come for HIV testing [and we have to say]. "Oh sorry we don't have the testing kits." Another day they come we test them. Like now we have female condoms; we don't have male condoms. Then we won't have female condoms; we will have male condoms. So it has been on and off throughout. (Interview, Zomba, June 28, 2011)

Just as was the case for community groups in Zambia that lost funding with the Global Fund–ZNAN scandal (see above), many Malawian groups widely reported their frustration with projects (FGDs and informal discussions, PLHIV groups, July–September 2011). And brokers, or those intermediaries between donors and local populations, reported on their own personal insecurity, including when they were not reimbursed for expenditures and services they provided (Informal discussions, NGO representatives, Lilongwe, Zomba, Karonga, Lusaka, and Ndola, March–September 2011).

This section has demonstrated the substantial cuts to aggregate funding in Malawi and the more targeted funding cuts in Zambia. In each case, PLHIV and PLHIV groups were impacted: ARVs became more difficult to acquire, community-level brokers lost funding, and AIDS projects ended. These cuts represented donors' more circumspect views of AIDS efforts in the two countries, particularly their concerns about corruption in the midst of the unprecedented amount of donor funding for health. And yet, while these cuts were detrimental, they also presented new opportunities for local agents, particularly in terms of extraversion and performances of compliance. Chapter 3 illustrates this dependent agency.

Sustainable Solutions and Local Empowerment

Another key change when we returned to Malawi and Zambia in 2011 was the shift among donors from an "emergency" AIDS response to one rooted in "sustainability" (See Swidler and Watkins 2009 on the sustainability doctrine that undergirds these projects; the doctrine assumes training and capital will enable local people to facilitate their own development.) One Zambian PLHIV said, "That phase [of providing immediate help] is already gone" (Interview, NZP+ leader, Mumbwa, April 15, 2011). The sustainability doctrine was evident in the Partnership Frameworks that PEPFAR signed with recipient countries in 2009, agreements intended to push country-owned sustainability plans that would incorporate civil society and increase the financial contributions from African governments to the AIDS response (PEPFAR 2013). The Malawian government also emphasized sustainability: "The new financing environment also means that the issue of sustainability and the coordination of the national response within national structures should be at the forefront of policy makers' thinking and actions" (GoM 2011, 10).

The on-the-ground outcome was that food distribution to PLHIV and AIDS orphans was scaled back, and donors sought to promote income-generation activities for PLHIV and caregivers. Donors gave loans to groups so they could start small enterprises (e.g., raising chickens, processing food, and making crafts to sell to tourists) or so that they could create savings and loan programs for their members. Trainings to engage in business and to manage such enterprises often accompanied the projects. For example, donors gave the NAPHAM support groups in Malawi farms, fertilizer, seeds, and revolving funds; they provided training through their "Pass-on" Project so participants could rear goats and "pass-on" their young to other groups. Donor officials asserted that because of widespread ART access in Zambia, many PLHIV were now healthy enough to "responsibly" take on their own development through "economic strengthening and self-help" (Interview, FBO official, Ndola, May 20, 2011; see also Kenworthy 2014). Echoing neoliberal sensibilities, one donor said, "We need to do a lot of mind-set changing in these groups. We need to tell them, 'Look, no one will feed you for the rest of your life. You really have to stand up and do for yourself'" (Interview, FBO official, Lusaka, March 31, 2011). The underlying logic of "empowering" local people to solve their own problems was widely invoked. An advocacy officer at NAPHAM, for example, reflected on how the focus should be to "build their capacity, give them the skills that they need and they will be the best agents of change" (Interview, Zomba, June 28, 2011).

The focus on sustainability was evident in our fieldwork. In Zambia, for example, 63 % of the PLHIV or caregiver groups we studied had done some income-generating activity, and an additional 20 % had a revolving loan program. Yet, these projects also reflected some of the challenges with the sustainability push in AIDS work, and the failure of the logic to not reflect on its own impact (Seckinelgin 2008, 1). One challenge was that such projects did not always succeed: of the Zambian groups, almost 40 % had experienced failed projects. Many group members described chickens that had died from disease or baskets that no one wanted to buy (Interview, PLHIV, Lusaka, March 1, 2011). Some of these project outcomes seemed unavoidable, but others resulted from mismanagement of group funds, free riders, or a lack of skills among members, all factors which the sustainability focus often discounts. In groups that had experienced problems with mismanagement, the morale was often low and participation, limited. When such negative outcomes emerged, the bias toward "stability" and "normal situations" which undergirds the push for sustainable projects may actually "produc[e] at best irrelevant and at worst damaging results for the survival strategies of the populations in the short as well as the long term" (De Bruijn and Van Dijk 1999, 6).

In this new environment, donors needed local groups and brokers to make sustainability work. Despite the aforementioned problems, donors often returned to the same local partners to implement projects. For example, over 50 % of church-based groups we studied in Zambia had experienced mismanagement, but most still had projects with international or Zambian FBOs. Donors' need to show results meant they turned to groups they knew, even if they might be inefficient (Interview, FBO official, Lusaka, March 31, 2011). However, as Chapter 4 points out, it was not always the case that local people recognized this action among donors. As Chapter 3 will further demonstrate, donors' move to a sustainable AIDS response and local empowerment opened various doors for dependent agency and necessitated brokers who could move across these lines between donors and recipients.

Dependent Agency Revisited

We have conceptualized that dependent agents like the PLHIV we studied demonstrate agency while situated in the tight corners of aid programs on which they depend. The poverty many of our research subjects faced meant they could not ignore donors' priorities and the Zambian and Malawian contexts highlight how local PLHIV and their associations were constrained by their limited opportunities. They often reacted when it came to donor initiatives: they formed groups in response to donors' need to institutionalize HIV testing and ARV dispersal; they developed income-generation projects when donors provided start-up capital and cut food distribution; and they suffered when each country was punished for high-level corruption scandals.

Yet the tight corners in which agents must maneuver are not static. The fluid donor landscape described in this chapter presented new opportunities for agents, particularly as the spaces expanded and contracted with shifts in donor funding and program focus. The projectified atmosphere with its multiple donors and local partners enabled dependent agents to move from group to group, searching resources. The changing preferences provided moments in which performances of compliance could occur and in which PLHIV could seek to redefine the issue. Donors' concerns about authenticity and sustainability, as well as their own dependence on local partners to achieve results, made agency possible. Thus, despite the fact that corruption scandals, funding cuts, and donors' focus on sustainability had the potential to disadvantage local PLHIV and their associations, some local PLHIV groups not only persevered, but they thrived, as the next chapter illustrates. (The final chapter acknowledges, however, that not all PLHIV benefited). We investigate the specific strategies that dependent agents used in this ever-changing context in the next chapter.

CHAPTER 3

Performing, Extraverting, and Resisting: The Strategies of Dependent Agents

Abstract This chapter analyzes strategies of dependent agents, using the empirical data and the works of James C. Scott and Jean-François Bayart. Performances of compliance echo donors' priorities and rhetoric. In extraversion, dependent agents outwardly highlight their dependency using testimonies and claims of donor exclusion. Donor-funded trainings are often the site for learning extraversion motifs and perfecting performances of compliance, and brokers, or people who link donors to community members, may facilitate this learning. Resistance below the line includes using euphemisms, stretching the rules, and foot-dragging. While dynamic, these strategies create leverage that facilitates access to opportunities and resources.

Keywords Strategies of dependent agents · Local responses · Performances of compliance · Extraversion · Resistance

A Malawian NGO representative in his early 30s invited one of the authors into his office in Zomba City for an interview with a welcoming smile. He was dressed in a purple shirt with a carefully fastened black tie embossed with a silver pattern; his flawless appearance stood somewhat in contrast to the office, which was almost empty save for the desk and chairs where he asked the author to sit. Behind his chair there was a noticeboard with a brightly colored HIV awareness calendar, a few documents from NAC, and a cut-out newspaper headline that read "AIDS fund rejection worries activists." As the interview began, he talked with enthusiasm about his role at the NGO and its work in the Zomba district. As he answered the author's questions, he demonstrated great confidence and expertise. Reflecting on the huge challenges he faced in his position and the issues that the NGO faced more generally, he remained positive about what could be achieved. At the end he offered the author some advice on her research plans and provided her with his business card.

Over the ensuing weeks the author and the NGO worker crossed paths on several occasions in Zomba City. He was always dressed in that same impeccable way with shoes that looked like they were shined that morning. He and the author also were often present at various stakeholder meetings and trainings, with the NGO worker representing his organization and claiming the various allowances for those events. It was not until a couple of weeks after the initial interview (and after several informal encounters), that the author learned that at the time she interviewed the NGO worker, his contract had ended because of NGO funding cuts. And yet, he continued to perform his role as leverage for personal opportunities, not least because he had a brother, cousin, and family friend for whom he was financially responsible. As he came to know the researcher, the NGO worker shared more critical insights into the NGO he had worked for and the broader HIV response in Zomba. Some of these points contradicted the answers he gave in the original interview.

These observations connect with this chapter's key issues about what dependent agency looks like within the context of structural poverty and aid dependence described in the previous chapter. We focus on local people acting as individuals or in community organizations who have been marginalized in the African politics and global health literatures (see Bayart 2000; Clapham 1996; Youde 2005; Brown 2014; Barnes et al. 2015). We investigate the way actors use performances as a form of leverage to access opportunities and resources. The above example illustrates that dependent agents may have multiple objectives: to gain resources to support kith and kin, to save face, and to maintain influence in the community. The example also shows changes in the actions of dependent agents, from holding an official, public position of a broker, to pretending to hold that position, to telling the back story about one's former position. Such dynamism is one theme of this chapter.

This chapter's goal is not to show the positive or negative effects of agency, such as its ability to change donor policies. We tackle this issue in

Chapter 4. Instead, we illustrate the multiple, and often overlapping, ways that local agents react to a donor context with high levels of resources and particular views of AIDS programs. We explore three strategies of agency. In the first, individuals and groups used what James C. Scott (1990) conceptualizes as *performances of compliance* with the intent of showing agreement with the "official story" (or public transcript) of the global health regime. Second, they utilized what Jean-François Bayart (2000) terms *extraversion*, often emphasizing their dependence, poverty, and marginalization in hopes of gaining more resources. Extraversion rarely challenges the official story, but rather plays upon and reifies outsiders' assumptions about the continent and AIDS in Africa. Finally, dependent agents utilized what Scott (1990, 198) refers to as *resistance below the line* or subversive reactions to the public transcript. In performances of compliance, extraversion, and resistance below the line, we find that *brokers*, or charismatic individuals who develop ties to external actors and local communities, played a crucial role as they translated objectives between recipients and donors and as they urged particular actions by local players. Our fieldwork in rural and urban Malawi and Zambia enables us to explore the dynamic and context-specific nature of agents' strategies, because we studied PLHIV groups that vary in duration, membership, and external support.

PERFORMANCES OF COMPLIANCE

In performances of compliance, dependent agents adopt specific phrases, behaviors, and structures that donors support. They learn and normalize the performances required of them, particularly through the technology of trainings. We use examples from more established PLHIV support groups to illustrate how some groups have perfected their performances over time. We contrast this "perfection" with actions in a Zambian group, which has had no reason to "learn the ropes." Yet because the powerful also are required to perform, local agents can use those official performances to point to hypocrisy.

Echoing the Official Story

As the observations in the chapter's introduction highlight, throughout the fieldwork the research participants performed for the authors. They widely echoed the rhetoric of donors and utilized the jargon of AIDS programs. As Chapter 1 highlighted, this AIDS narrative stresses that AIDS is an exceptional disease that requires an exceptional response, one which must protect human rights and include PLHIV in policymaking, advocacy, and service delivery. PLHIV must be empowered so that the AIDS response is sustainable. Rooted in neoliberal assumptions about individual autonomy, the official story assumes that information, training, and income-generating projects will facilitate empowerment. Health education and disclosure of one's HIV status in open and transparent ways are crucial (Nguyen 2010; Benton 2015).

There were several overlapping ways that individual PLHIV and PLHIV groups "bought into" this public AIDS transcript. First, they adopted particular labels and vocabularies that donors utilized. Some identified as "activists," a moniker that many Africans avoid because it connotes an adversarial stance toward the state rather than a willingness to build consensus; in short, activists are "controversial" (Ellis and van Kessel 2009; Interview, NGO official, Lusaka, April 15, 2009). Yet donors viewed activism positively because it had led to access to AIDS medications and services for PLHIV, and they viewed organizations such as the AIDS Coalition to Unleash Power (ACT UP) in the United States and the Treatment Action Campaign (TAC) in South Africa as models for advocacy (Johnson 2006; Kapstein and Busby 2013; Gould 2009). Donors sought to join forces with local PLHIV "activist" groups, such as when the international NGO Action Aid teamed up with the COWLHA to promote the rights of women living with HIV (WLHIV) (Interview, Action Aid official, Lilongwe, July 17, 2007).

Thus emphasizing one's activism could be a strategic choice, as the following dialogue with a local PLHIV illustrates:

Interviewer: Do you call yourself an activist?
Respondent: Yes, yes, of course.
Interviewer: Have you been criticized for being an activist?
Respondent: Of course. From my family, but now they are seeing what has been coming out of my activism. They have been assisted and now they are coming on board. At the beginning, yes, I was exiled. But not now. They even want more activists in the family.

The respondent explained that because he was an activist he was invited to workshops (which gave per diems), he was once interviewed on television, and he had received small stipends from NGOs for his volunteer work. In a telling conclusion, the interviewee dashed off to a meeting of activists linked to a Zambian NGO that works on legal discrimination for PLHIV and that had received donor funding for human rights education (Interview, NZP+ official, Lusaka, May 10, 2011).

Church groups also performed, using religious imagery and biblical verses when they interacted with international FBOs. One Zambian FBO explained that its objective as a Christian group working on AIDS was to "be the salt and light" in God's kingdom; it hoped to show God's love through its AIDS work and to bring PLHIV to Christ (Interview, FBO official, Ndola, May 20, 2011; see Matthew 5: 13–16). One of its caregivers echoed this evangelical theme: "Our own faith has grown because of our work with AIDS orphans and people suffering" (FGD, caregiving group, Ndola, May 21, 2011). This rhetoric resonated with the FBO's Western partners, many of whom were evangelical churches (Interview, FBO partner, Minneapolis, MN, August 21, 2013).

Similarly, in a meeting of 18 Malawian stakeholders from local NGOs, attendees strategized about how to comply with donor requirements, particularly by using such donor-preferred terms as "coordination," "cooperation," "negotiation," "inclusiveness," "comprehensive coverage," "shared responsibility," and "consensus" (Participant observation, stakeholders' meeting, Zomba City, July 5, 2011). Donors' jargon was also evident in support groups' talk about "living positively" (or alternatively, "positive living"). Members of one Malawian group, for example, presented themselves as positively embracing their HIV status: "We are free to tell people we are HIV positive; we are free to shout it out" (FGD, PLHIV group, Makunganya, Zomba, July 29, 2011). It is possible they made these claims to appeal to donors and the author, perhaps in this instance because the group was not registered with NAPHAM, the gatekeeper for much funding.

A second way we saw performances of compliance was through behavior, specifically the reported adoption of activities associated with "positive living," such as getting tested for HIV, urging others to be tested, and disclosing one's HIV status. In FGDs, many participants enthusiastically supported these actions: they said they were fortunate to know their HIV status because they had tested for HIV. One Zambian woman explained, "In lots of groups there are people who are HIV positive and HIV negative. But the difference is that we know our status" (FGD, PLHIV group, Lusaka, March 22, 2011). This knowledge empowered members: "We know our status and we are on medication. We may very well live longer than the people who don't know their status" (FGD, PLHIV group, Lusaka, March 24, 2011). PLHIV often pointed out that knowledge was beneficial: "We are happy, because we have a lot of information, even if the community laughs at us. They don't know what they talk about" (FGD, PLHIV group, Kitwe, May 19, 2011). In a performance to one of the researchers and NGO officials, a Malawian organization highlighted the members' adoption of positive living:

> The [PLHIV] group helps them [the members] because their worries go away. We remind each other about what we hear at the testing clinic, give testimony to others (about our status) to encourage others. We encourage those taking drugs to tell their partners (a lot of people are not transparent) and advocate for HIV tests. We encourage abstinence because we belong to the church. We encourage HIV counseling to our peers. We have tried to reach out a lot and we do individual outreach but we are planning to have group outreach. We have so far consulted the chief to organize an outreach and it worked. (Participant observation, caregiver group, Zomba, July 13, 2011)

In the presence of donors, the researchers, and NGO officials, not only did many groups proudly discuss how they met the obligations of positive living, but they also pointed out when some individuals had not met such expectations. Some PLHIV reported that other PLHIV drank alcohol excessively or had sex without using a condom (Informal conversation, NZP+ leader, Lusaka, March 24, 2011). Several PLHIV groups criticized caregivers because they had not been tested for HIV, thus implying that caregivers had not lived up to the official AIDS transcript (FGDs, PLHIV groups, Lusaka, March 8–10, 2011). Many of the groups that made such accusations had not received donor money while the HBC groups had. The PLHIV complaints appeared to have little traction with donors, potentially because the official story about HBC stressed caregivers' compassion, generosity, and willingness to give their time and energy to PLHIV; it did not emphasize caregivers' own HIV status (Maes 2014).

Because local agents have been exposed to the same donor jargon, images, and ideals in different countries, we heard many of the same phrases in performances in both countries. In addition to "positive living", we often encountered the word "free", which connoted freedom from the AIDS stigma, access to information, and autonomy in choices. One Zambian PLHIV explained: "Now [after being in the group] I am with a free mind. Previously I used to think that the only resort for me is death. But from the group, I have information and I am now very free" (FGD, PLHIV group,

Lusaka, March 22, 2011). Female group members (and some males) often said women were "free" including with respect to negotiating sex with their husbands (FGDs, PLHIV groups, Fulirwa, Karonga, September 2, 2011 and Lusaka, March 24, 2011). We do not doubt these sentiments, because the dominated may accept the official transcript. Rather we stress the common use of these transcripts, particularly when donors (and researchers) were present.

A third performance of compliance was to adopt donor-approved structures, particularly PLHIV groups which, in turn, had been crucial in AIDS advocacy and service delivery in the West (Gould 2009; Nguyen 2010). The PLHIV group became an arena in which to practice performances of compliance. Sometimes, though, this meant "making a group" when none really existed. For example, one author was taken to meet a "new" PLHIV group in Zambia. During the FGD, it became apparent that the members had never worked together: they shared no stories of common experiences, they sat apart from one another, and they did not converse before or after the meeting. When the author later asked her informant about the group's behavior, she was told, "They thought you were bringing something and they showed up." Because they knew that "donors like support groups," they performed "being a group" (Participant observation, PLHIV group, Lusaka, March 30, 2011).

As a technology of agency, adoption of donor-preferred structures also included setting up formal rules, electing officials, writing bylaws, recording meeting minutes, and writing (and submitting) reports. As Watkins and Swidler (2013, 207) explain, "Every CBO in Malawi has a standard array of committees corresponding to donor themes (OVC, Home Based Care, PLWA [Persons Living with AIDS], Youth), each with an executive committee, and all must submit regular reports to their funder." Structural transformation also could mean affiliation with a larger network like NZP+ or NAPHAM, groups which often acted as gatekeepers to donor funding. For example, one Zambian group that affiliated with NZP+ had only seven members, all from two families. But the group linked to NZP+ was created "because we needed technical assistance and connections" which it hoped NZP+ would bring. To show its "official" status, it adopted elections, bylaws, and a regular meeting schedule (FDG, PLHIV group, Lusaka, March 24, 2011).

We repeatedly observed an underlying dynamic in performances: respondents utilized different "on stage" and "off stage" scripts (see Scott 1990, 16). Frustrated with donor-funding cuts and reshuffled priorities for AIDS programs, in informal conversations a number of respondents expressed opinions or acted in ways that would be at odds with the official story they presented in formal interviews. For example, at the district-level offices of NGOs in Zomba City, the key informant interviewees dressed formally, officially represented their NGOs, and talked enthusiastically about their projects and their professional life. Yet in later informal discussions, a number of them revealed that they were actually at the end of their contracts, that they had already officially lost their positions, or that their projects had not been operating for a long time. The individual in this chapter's introduction said he dressed each day for work despite the end of his contract so that others in Zomba City would take him seriously. This performance enabled him to continue receiving payments for attending training sessions and meetings as a representative of the NGO. His initial performance for the author was perhaps in part a strategy to leverage his position for potential opportunities that the author may offer (Informal discussions, NGO representatives, Zomba, July 2011).

Brokers used these onstage and offstage scripts. As local "big men," brokers are expected to ensure the general survival of all those in their patronage networks such as extended family, friends, and community members; they must distribute aid, wealth, and food just as a father is expected to provide for his family (Hyden 2006; De Smedt 2009; Schratzberg 2001). To meet this role (or to appear to meet it), during FGDs, brokers praised the groups' project successes, asserted that group members cared for one another, and positively assessed the members' hard work. Yet once out of the public eye (e.g., on the drive home), these intermediaries said very different things. In one instance, an NZP+ district coordinator said the just-interviewed group was controversial and poorly run; in another example, an FBO broker ranted about how one group had misused funds and its leadership was not transparent (Informal conversations, NZP+ leader, Lusaka, June 10, 2011 and FBO coordinator, Kitwe, May 22, 2011). Even though they knew that the author had no resources, during the FGDs, these individuals performed for the local group because part of their responsibility as patrons was to showcase these groups' strengths. But because the position of brokers is vulnerable (see Lewis and Mosse 2006), these intermediaries also needed to give the authors "inside information," thus making themselves indispensable. The on- and offstage rhetoric shows that performances of compliance are not static and that brokers adapt to different audiences.

Learning and Normalizing the Required Performances

Performances had to be learned, and that process often occurred in physical spaces and temporal moments. Church groups, for example, utilized the church building for meetings because it was often provided at no charge and was centrally located, and these groups capitalized on denominationally mandated events like "AIDS recognition Sunday" or "women's Sunday" to publicize specific rhetoric and images (Interview, FBO official, Lusaka, April 1, 2011; Participant observation, church service, Lusaka, August 5, 2007). Similarly, AIDS clinics were a venue where PLHIV interacted with other PLHIV, volunteers, and paid clinic workers, some of whom acted as brokers to donor-funded programs. Because PLHIV often had to spend long hours at clinics, and because they had to visit clinics regularly to obtain their medications, these spaces were ideal for learning the official AIDS transcript (Whyte et al. 2013; Participant observations, AIDS clinic, Lusaka, March 9–13, 2011).

But perhaps the most crucial arena in which local people learned AIDS performances was the training sessions. These are extensively conducted in local communities because they "make everyone happy" by appealing to norms of sustainability and by providing participants with per diems, transport funds, and food and drinks for the day (Watkins and Swidler 2013, 207; Smith 2003). For example, a female trainee in Malawi explicitly stated after a training session that a main benefit of NGOs is that "they give us food like today—Fanta, bananas" (FGD, PLHIV group, Kasowa, Karonga, August 22, 2011). Trainings were extensively promoted in Malawi and Zambia, and our empirical research indicates that they led to the adoption of a common language for performances.

To illustrate the learning of performances, we use the example of NAPHAM, a major organization conducting training sessions with PLHIV nationwide in Malawi. Despite donors' broader retraction of funds, NAPHAM extended its programs to all 28 districts in 2011. It also established a district office in Zomba City in February 2011 and by June, 103 support groups with over 7000 members had been registered (Interview, NAPHAM coordinator, Zomba, June 28, 2011). NAPHAM provided training sessions to empower and strengthen these groups in the areas of HIV education outreach, group therapy, youth and child therapy, psychosocial support, counseling and guidance, leadership, report writing, and financial management. Through the process of HIV education outreach, NAPHAM staff identified groups with high potential for learning and then selected both male and female group members to be trained. Once trained, representatives were supposed to share what they had learned with group members in the district (Interview, NAPHAM official, Lilongwe, June 16, 2011).

In June 2011, 28 people (half men and half women) who were from 14 newly registered support groups attended the first district-level training sessions about group therapy. During the training sessions one of the authors observed how the participants learned and normalized particular performances. The training sessions were very participatory, and they helped to establish norms of behavior and schedules and structures for individual support group meetings. The training sessions were designed to "ensure there is some guidance for what they should discuss and advise the members of their support groups" (Interview, NAPHAM coordinator, Zomba, June 28, 2011). The participants engaged in discussions about how they understood issues that PLHIV groups face, role-plays about how to support other PLHIV, and singing and dancing to help facilitate memorization of certain lessons. In the "Positive Living" lesson on psychological and physical well-being, participants were invited to sit inside the ring of tables and to share their own ideas and experiences. This exercise highlighted the importance of disclosure and openness, while also allowing the PLHIV to show off for the other attendees. Throughout the training, the participants learned through repetition and were praised when they correctly performed the required actions or gave the required responses (Participant observation, NAPHAM trainings, Zomba City, June 27–29, 2011). Trainees also performed for potential gatekeepers to resources who facilitated or observed parts of the sessions, since trainings were a "honeypot" that attracted individuals such as NAPHAM representatives, government health officials, representatives from NGOs and FBOs, private philanthropists, and one author. All of these individuals could be potential benefactors.

We were curious about how lessons learned trickled down to local PLHIV groups after the trainings. Following the NAPHAM training, one author was invited to several support group meetings, and a week later, she attended one meeting in Nsondole. This was the first group meeting following the trainings, and the chairperson was reporting back from the sessions. At the training, the chairperson had appeared to be particularly engaged and responsive to the lessons learned. Indeed he had approached the author to invite her to his support group. However, his communication with the group about what he learned was limited to quickly mentioning that he went to the training and noting that "they learnt a lot and there will be some few changes. Now I am no master of ceremony but will be the group therapy leader." He highlighted just one idea from the training for his group: "Whilst at the training we saw a suggestion box—that is the need for any member to throw any worry that he/she has, so everyone is encouraged to suggest in the group" (Participant observation, PLHIV group, Nsondole, Zomba, July 6, 2011). Thus while participants learn to perform for donors at training sessions, they may not transfer many concrete lessons from training sessions to others (see also Watkins and Swidler 2013).

Yet, even if trainees shared little specific knowledge from trainings, they did bring home exposure to the expected jargon, behaviors, structures, and stories of the official AIDS transcript. Trainees seemed to share these bigger messages, as evident in a newly formed NZP+ group. One trained group leader explained the "rules" for structuring the group: "Every group should have five to 15 in a group, otherwise it is too hard to organize. Maybe 20. . . . If there are 40 or 50 interested, then form another group. Each group needs a chairperson and then it needs committees: a psychological committee, livelihood committee, IEC [information and education committee] and a social committee." The new organization's members nodded dutifully. And when one woman referred to members as "people with AIDS," she was quickly corrected by another trained leader. "Let's not say 'AIDS' for that means death. We are people with HIV." He then asked the group to repeat three times, "We are people with HIV." In the process, the group learned the accepted structures and words used in performances of compliance (Participant observation, PLHIV group, Lusaka, May 5, 2011).

Despite the ambiguous benefits of trainings, both new and well-established support groups in both countries wanted these opportunities. At the same time, many of these groups were fairly critical of the limitations of the training they had already received. For example, the chairperson of the HBC group in Zomba City explained, "We need trainings to empower us—counseling alone is not enough—so that when we meet we benefit a lot. The aim of the group is to make these people live a long life" (Participant observations and FDGs, PLHIV groups, Zomba City, Zomba, July 27, 2011). Similarly, a long-standing church HBC group in Lusaka demanded more trainings, despite the fact that since its establishment in 2002, it had "participated in seminars, trainings, and had benefited from workshops." The group bemoaned the fact that "there are no trainings now like in the past" (FGD, caregiver group, Lusaka, April 7, 2011). As we indicate below, pleas for trainings were a crucial aspect of extraversion strategies, since they brought material benefits. Yet in keeping with the performance of compliance, during the FGDs, local actors discussed the knowledge benefits, expertise, and skills they gained at trainings, and not these material perks. One Zambian PLHIV said, "I have gained so much health information, and I have shared [it] with my wife, my children, and people in my church so we can all be safe from HIV" (Interview, Lusaka, May 10, 2011).

Brokers played a large role in determining who did (or did not) attend trainings. In Malawi, one NAPHAM district coordinator explained this gatekeeper role:

> There is no faith-based organization or community-based organization that can get funding without the reference of NAPHAM. They have been trying and write nice proposals to convince people. But NAC comes to NAPHAM and asks, "Have you trained them on anything on HIV?" They want a reference. Do we think they have capacity? [In the past] the money was not reaching the right people. (Interview, NAPHAM Coordinator, Zomba, June 28, 2011)

Similarly, NZP+ district coordinators often helped to choose individuals from specific support groups to attend trainings, in order to reach the "right people" (Interview, NZP+ leader, Kabwe, April 18, 2011). While this process limited group infighting, it increased the power of these intermediaries. Yet brokers' power was tenuous, since money for trainings could dry up, as occurred when NAPHAM lost funds partway through its training program in Zomba and had to put district-level trainings on hold indefinitely.

Perfecting the Performances of Compliance

Given the situations of extreme dependency in Malawi and Zambia, over time people learned what hoops they needed to jump through, including the jargon, behaviors, and structures they must adopt and the specific requirements they must fulfil in writing proposals, log frames, and reports (see DiMaggio and Powell 1983). Because these performances are dynamic, it is useful to compare older PLHIV organizations that have had time to perfect performances with more recently formed groups. More established groups included NAPHAM groups in Karonga district, Malawi (established in 2008), and one NZP+ group in Livingstone, Zambia (established in 2004). The Karonga and Livingstone groups had adapted themselves to meet donors' shifting requirements, even redefining themselves when necessary. As evidence, the men in one Karonga group created a CBO to meet donors' funding requirements after they lost NAC funding (FGD, PLHIV group, Nyungwe, Karonga, August 27, 2011). Another Karonga group performed perfectly at a NGO-led review exercise on nutrition that one author observed. The participants sat upright and attentively, appearing to participate enthusiastically, providing what were seemingly the "right answers" in follow-up questions, and self-reporting that they had changed their health and sexual behavior because of their HIV status. They had learned that perfected performances were necessary because sometimes development actors play communities against one another. At the training, the HIV coordinator made it explicit that "there are 20 groups that want to be trained but we will work with eight only." This competitive environment made trainings and review exercises crucial tools that funders used to assess these groups' knowledge about and commitment to HIV and AIDS, since they could observe how well group members had memorized lessons and hear reports on group activities (Participant observation, NGO training group, Kasowa, Karonga, August 22, 2011).

And yet, once the NGO representatives departed from this specific training, the performance masks came off and the atmosphere changed. During informal discussions, issues emerged relating to diet and nutrition. One woman questioned why she was losing so much weight and her ARVs were not working. After some teasing from her husband and the other group members it transpired that, despite her answers during the NGO assessment and her initial appeals, she was not eating a balanced diet or drinking enough water while taking her ARVs because she preferred to just eat *nsima* and drink Fanta (Participant observation, PLHIV group, Kasowa, Karonga, August 22, 2011).[1] Thus, while she could perform the right answers, she had not internalized them in terms of her own behavior.

The Livingstone group went beyond adopting approved PLHIV group structures or repeating lessons learned at trainings in its perfected performances, though it did those things too. It also developed a highly organized money-making partnership in collaboration with an international hotel that catered to tourists, a project that epitomized donors' neoliberal aspirations for sustainability. The group raised worms which ate the hotel's food refuse and, as a result, created waste fertilizer that was spread on the hotel's gardens. Group members "fed" the worms and collected the fertilizer. The group had an elaborate work schedule and over time, it had made enough money to set up two bank accounts (one for the project and another to pay for members' emergencies). In its performance, the group stressed this sustainable project led by committed, local men and women. One member said, "We are progressing, progressing. We are a dynamic group and I think we are the only group in Livingstone...which has sustained a long run project for some time. We have a lot of members...Through our own contributions we have been able to work hard...And we have learned so much" (FGD, PLHIV group, Livingstone, June 27, 2011). Members enthusiastically spoke of other accomplishments too, including the development of a school for AIDS orphans and the physical health of most members. While we recognize these accomplishments, we also assert that the group engaged in a performance that emphasized neoliberal sentiments about self-empowerment. It also downplayed some of its challenges, such as members who "forgot" about their worm-farm chores. As part of an offstage script, these challenges only emerged during informal discussions as the researcher was preparing to leave (FGD, PLHIV group, Livingstone, June 27, 2011).

Not all groups had perfected these performances. Some were newly established and had not had sufficient time to learn, as was the case for some groups in Zomba District. But others seemed to have decided that performances brought few (if any) benefits. For example, NGOs that had promised to assist one Lusaka group had not done so and the prior president had stolen all of the group's funds. The group was highly skeptical of outsiders, and as a result, on the day of a planned FGD, only the president and two officers showed up. Highly embarrassed, the president made numerous excuses: people were working, there was a funeral, some were sick (FGD, PLHIV, Lusaka, April 14, 2011). While nonattendance could have been the result of other factors (e.g., poor group communication), it was notable that of all 57 FGDs conducted with PLHIV in Zambia, this was the only one with such weak attendance. Thus, the group's prior experiences destroyed any incentive to perform for outsiders.

Official Transcripts Cut Both Ways: Holding Powerful Actors to Account

The performances of the dominant are necessary to support their claims to legitimacy (Scott 1990, 10). When the actions of powerful partners (in our case, donors) do not resonate with the public transcript, dependent agents can use this disconnect as leverage by charging hypocrisy. As Chapter 1 illustrated, donors had emphasized human rights norms and, in some cases, religious values that undergird access to ART, food, and AIDS programs. They also had stressed nondiscrimination as a crucial norm in the AIDS fight. These themes were evident in trainings; for example, one Zambian FBO stressed that access to treatment and PLHIV empowerment are ways to show God's love for his people (Interview, FBO trainee, Ndola, June 6, 2014). In both countries, local groups pointed out how donors' actions often did not align with these official transcripts. In Malawi, one group reported that the Ministry of Agriculture had not provided it with an engine (Participant observation, NAPHAM executive meeting, Karonga Boma, August 19, 2011). In Zambia, one group member said, "There was this [NGO], and they wanted to assist us with loans for projects. But they never assisted us, even after two weeks of trainings. They did not give us loans" (Interview, PLHIV, Lusaka, March 1, 2011). Sometimes these complaints highlighted how donors preferred select community members, a practice that violated the ideal of nondiscrimination. In Malawi, one support group said that a Canadian NGO had only been interested in women (Participant observation, NAPHAM executive meeting, Karonga Boma, August 19, 2011), and a Zambian church PLHIV group complained that FBOs only supported HBC groups, never PLHIV groups (FGD, PLHIV group, Lusaka, March 9, 2011).

Lack of access to ART was a powerful theme in these complaints, because it cut into the heart of donors' motivation to develop PEPFAR and the Global Fund. Chapter 2 showed that funding cuts meant that not all individuals gained access to ARVs or that some PLHIV received their medications on an erratic schedule. AIDS activists used donors' own vocabulary of human rights when funding cuts curtailed ART availability, and they also played up the discourse of "Africa as a victim of the West." For example, after the Global Fund scandal in Zambia one activist said, "There are people out there who don't even know the Global Fund money was stolen, but who depend on it. They go to the facility, are told there is no treatment, and they have no idea why. But they are Zambians, and they have a right to treatment" (*IRIN News*,

March 14, 2011). The speaker highlights the "right" to treatment, echoing the norm that donors had stressed, as well as building an image of an innocent and uninformed PLHIV who is at the mercy of government corruption and global forces. The human right to treatment was apparent when activists complained about ART access in rural areas, where populations were very isolated due to poor roads and high transportation costs. One Zambian PLHIV group leader said that donors and the government needed to live up to their promises for treatment access and help rural people (Interview, PLHIV, Mpika, July 4, 2011). The interviewee pointed to the hypocrisy in donors' inaction.

Food distribution was another topic for charges of hypocrisy, as well as strategies of extraversion (see below). In terms of hypocrisy, groups pointed out that donors had been more than willing to give out food when they needed people to test for HIV. They had led people to believe that food would always be available to PLHIV. One woman said, "How could they do one thing and then, they change their minds? While they are changing their priorities, we are hungry. Don't they care?" (Interview, PLHIV, Lusaka, March 8, 2011).

Christian values of compassion for people who are suffering and biblical demands to serve the hungry, ill, impoverished, and lonely could emerge in hypocrisy charges too. FBOs had stressed that caregivers who helped PLHIV and/or AIDS orphans were generous, committed Christians who engaged in physically exhausting and, sometimes, financially costly work. For these FBO representatives, caregivers lived out the biblical mandate to love one's neighbor as oneself (Interview, FBO official, Lusaka, April 15, 2007; see also Vander Meulen et al. 2013; Root and van Wyngaard 2011). Yet caregivers often pointed out that Christian compassion did not seem to extend to them. They too were hungry, tired, and poor. One said, "They [donors] always say the PLHIV are vulnerable, but we too are vulnerable ones" (FGD, caregivers, Kitwe, May 19, 2011).

Two general patterns of hypocrisy charges were evident. First, if many donors worked in an area, the support groups and CBOs could use hypocrisy claims to play one donor against another. The FGDs revealed that support groups and CBOs in Zomba and Karonga in Malawi, as well as Lusaka, Kitwe, Kabwe, and Livingstone in Zambia, were very knowledgeable about the organizations working in their areas and what each one offered. In one Malawian support group, for example, men reported that they worked with several NGOs: one NGO established a project, another provided fertilizer and condoms to PLHIV, another provided counseling and guidance on producing nutritious foods, and another gave porridge. Comparing the donors, the group was critical of one NGO because it had yet to do anything with them, despite being there for two months (FGD, PLHIV group, Nsondole, Zomba, August 3, 2011). A second pattern was that support groups with longer histories (such as those in Karonga district) were more likely to point to donors' hypocrisy. These groups were more confident in their autonomy, resources, and leadership (FGDs and observations, PLHIV groups, Zomba, Karonga, Livingstone, and Kitwe, May–September, 2011). These patterns illustrated changes in time and group development.

This section has demonstrated how dependent agents engage in performances of compliance, adopting the technologies of jargon (e.g., positive living and activism) as well as donor-approved practices (e.g., PLHIV group rules and responsible PLHIV behavior) in order to garner favor with donors, NGO partners, and researchers. Trainings or physical spaces like churches or AIDS clinics were venues in which the vocabularies and images needed in performances could spread, and brokers helped local people to learn such technologies and perfect such practices. The uncertainty of AIDS funding in both countries, as well as donors' own norms, provided opportunities for using these strategies to point to donors' hypocrisy.

Extraversion

In the context of shifting donor priorities and funding cuts, extraversion enabled individuals and groups to use their weaknesses and to play upon predominant views of Africa in the West in order to gain resources. NGOs encouraged support groups to mobilize their situations for funding and support. For example, at a NAPHAM executive meeting, the district coordinator urged all support group representatives to engage in extraversion, saying, "We need lots of things as Karonga District. Please think to ask people wherever you are going. I have the hope that whatever you find in your groups, you will link them to others who need help" (Participant observation, NAPHAM executive meeting, Karonga Boma, August 19, 2011). Sometimes this "asking" seemed like little more than a laundry list of requests to donors, NGOs workers, and even the researchers. For example, one Fulirwa support group member said, "We want an office," to which other group members added, "a modern one—we have built a traditional one." Another added that they needed transport for outreach and training on group therapy. The first member concluded, "We do not receive any *chiponde*" (FGD, PLHIV group, Fulirwa, Karonga, September 2, 2011).[2]

We investigate such "asking," by exploring five extraversion themes we encountered: the diseased body, the marginalized PLHIV, the entrepreneurial woman, the healthy, empowered (and often, grateful) PLHIV, and the authentic PLHIV support group. We then question how dependent agents may use development actors' practices and priorities as themes for extraversion. Extraversion is used to get access to trainings, which, in turn, become a major arena in which extraversion is learned. Throughout these processes, brokers play an important role in translating between the dominant party (e.g., donors) and local organizations.

Extraversion around PLHIV Testimonies

The outward process whereby people extraverted their diseased bodies— or *became* HIV-positive peoples (see Igoe 2006)—was a fundamental strategy for survival and even upward social mobility in Malawi and Zambia. *Becoming* HIV-positive people required PLHIV to give testimonials about their own personal history with HIV. As indicated above, donors themselves have emphasized the testimony as part of the therapy process (Nguyen 2010; Benton 2015). As this book's opening observation indicated, the authors were approached within and outside of the formal research process by individuals who wanted to tell their AIDS stories (Interviews, FGDs, and informal discussions, Lusaka, Kabwe, Kitwe, Lilongwe, Zomba, and Karonga, April–September, 2011). These stories had several overlapping themes. The first emphasized the diseased body, particularly the ravages that AIDS and, sometimes, ART itself brought to the PLHIV. For example, a Zambian PLHIV spoke at length about how ART made him so dizzy he could not work to feed his family (Interview, PLHIV, Lusaka, March 2, 2011). Another Zambian PLHIV who was visibly ill at one AIDS clinic insisted on meeting with a researcher to detail her cough, fever, and weakness (Interview, PLHIV, Lusaka, March 1, 2011). Such images fit with Western perceptions of AIDS as a crisis and emergency.

The diseased body theme often linked to a second theme: the poverty and marginalization of PLHIV. In these scenarios, AIDS was sometimes "paraded" for donors (and researchers) to encounter, with particular groups showcased as the public face of PLHIV marginalization. For example, one family of HIV-positive orphans was showcased at NAPHAM trainings in Zomba City; they were photographed and given clothing and support for their school fees (Participant observation, NAPHAM trainings, Zomba City, June 27–29, 2011). Similarly, five AIDS orphans in Zambia were brought to a FGD, though the researcher did not request their presence. The children sat politely and dutifully, while the group leader pointed to each and said,

> This one, both parents are dead. That one is on treatment. That one, the father is dead and the mother is still around, though she is doing nothing. And those two: that one, the mother is dead and the father is around, and the other, the father is dead. And even if the parents are still living, they are unemployed, struggling. And just to add, that girl, her parents are dead. It is like her family, they don't care for her. And all of them, the group is in charge of taking care of them and getting their medications. (FGD, PLHIV group, Lusaka, March 23, 2011)

While the children were clearly impoverished, the showcasing of these children aligned with many donors' emphasis on AIDS orphans (Hunter and Wilkinson 1997; Interviews, International NGOs and FBOs, Lusaka, August 5–18, 2007). The children (and their plight) became a resource for PLHIV groups, who referred to them as "their children" or "their groups," and to themselves as the children's custodians (Participant observation, NAPHAM trainings, Zomba City, June 27–29, 2011). As gatekeepers, they used extraversion stories to negotiate potential access to the children for external actors.

A third extraversion theme among PLHIV related to gender, including both women's vulnerability to HIV and their entrepreneurial response to the disease. AIDS experts, policymakers, and scholars have stressed the political, economic, and sociocultural reasons African women are vulnerable to HIV (See Baylies and Bujra 2000; Anderson 2012, 2015; Siplon and Novotny 2007). We found in both countries that women often highlighted these themes in FGDs. In one all-women PLHIV group, members said, "We are just women, mothers, widows; we have nothing in this community" (FGD, PLHIV group, Lusaka, March 24, 2011), a statement that implied their need for external help. In one Malawian group meeting, women gave several gendered reasons that HIV was high in their area. One said, "Polygamy—my husband and the young wife were HIV positive, and then in 2008 I was also tested positive. On May 18, 2008 I started ARVs and now no sickness. I am very healthy." A second woman explained, "*Fisi* because of my parents who forced me,"[3] while a third woman offered that "it went into my family before I had a blood test." Even some men highlighted gendered practices as increasing HIV vulnerability: "I was tested positive in 2006 because of polygamy and other concubines" (Participant observation, PLHIV group, Nsondole, Zomba, July 6, 2011). We recognize that these practices increase women's vulnerability to HIV: our point is that discussion of these cultural and social practices became a resource for extraversion.

Development projects have typically targeted women, because economic and cultural structures tend toward gendered inequalities in land distribution (both in terms of the customary and modern systems of land inheritance), agriculture, food security, and labor opportunities. The majority of Zambian and Malawian women are relatively poor within the family unit and are financially dependent upon their husbands for their own and their children's survival, especially in the rural areas where poverty is more acute (Baylies and Bujra 2000). Women's dependence was particularly high in patrilineal systems (such as those of Karonga district or among the Bemba in northern Zambia), because the wife moves to the husband's village, land is inherited through the man's lineage, and women access land through their husbands. Men dominate the family and the woman's father or husband is the highest authority (see Anderson 2015; Peters 1992).

Despite these obstacles, many respondents said that women are "entrepreneurial." Their initiative taking, as well as their marginalization in society, urges donors to provide them with loans, projects (like raising chickens or gardening), training for the projects, and inputs (Interviews, FBO and NGO officials, Lusaka, August 2007, February and March 2011). In fact, the aforementioned Zambian group of "only widows" had a very successful chick raising project, the profits from which were used to help members with emergency expenses like medications for sick children or funeral costs (FGD, PLHIV group, Lusaka, March 24, 2011).

While some women could use their gendered marginalization and perceived entrepreneurial spirit to their advantage, men were less successful in playing to these extraversion narratives. Instead, it was often assumed that the majority of men only came to PLHIV activities in search of immediate benefits. While men have more alternative options for income generation, they also are less likely to join support groups (see Patterson 2015). One respondent explained: "Men do not want to [be as open as women about their HIV status]. Men say it was my wife that brought the virus. They are the breadwinners. They do not like to participate in groups like these where they don't get anything. They would rather go to work to earn something" (Interview, NAPHAM coordinator, Zomba, June 28, 2011; see also interview, AIDS clinic counsellor, Lusaka, March 2, 2011).

Despite men's hesitancy to participate in PLHIV activities, high poverty and unemployment rates meant that men were increasingly unable to fulfill heir gender-based roles as providers (Anderson 2015, 118–119; on South Africa see Seekings and Nattrass 2005). They too increasingly looked for ways to use dependence and marginalization to achieve benefits (see Ferguson 2013, 231). For example, in Zomba district, some men were presenting themselves as men who have sex with men (MSM) to gain access to new donor projects that targeted those subpopulations, even though in Malawi (and Zambia) homosexuality is illegal and stigmatized. These individuals even presented themselves or their friends as MSM to one author with the hope that she could link them to opportunities for assistance (Interviews, informal discussions, and observations, Zomba district, July–August, 2011). Despite these attempts, men also found that their extraversion efforts lacked an audience, for they did not resonate with donors' perceptions that men tend to be the partner who brings HIV into a relationship or that men have economic opportunities. Men are rarely perceived to be individuals who are vulnerable or marginalized (see Aggleton et al. 2014). As a result, donor projects continued to disproportionately benefit women. As one Malawian man explained, small loans were available to women to start small businesses like selling baked goods, but there were no reasonable loans for men to start larger businesses (Interview, NGO representative, Zomba, July 22, 2011).

In addition, extraversion could emphasize how biomedicine and self-empowerment led to PLHIV's transformation. For example, at a training session of MANET+ in Mponela, Malawi, a PLHIV shared her testimony with one author. She reflected that when she was diagnosed as HIV positive in 2000, she was prepared to pay MWK 5000 a month for ARVs but these drugs were not available in the private or government clinics. A few pilot projects were distributing ARVs but only to those people in select districts. The woman initially experienced high levels of discrimination when she went out of her house: people pointed and called her a "walking corpse" and "skeleton" when she traveled on the bus to the Queen Elizabeth Hospital in Blantyre to try to find ARVs.

When she managed to access drugs illegally from South Africa through family connections, her health improved. Over time, she was asked to join networks for PLHIV, and she used her identity as a WLHIV to access opportunities to represent WLHIV at international conferences and to visit other countries (Informal discussion, WLHIV, Mponela, June 26, 2011). Biomedicine and empowerment through the AIDS enterprise itself led to personal transformation, and her PLHIV identity opened the doors to these opportunities.

In a second example, a PLHIV working with a Zambian NGO explained how he started ARVs quite late, "when I was about dead." Then his wife left him, taking their two children: "She packed up everything, even bringing a truck to get things. We had even had a church wedding and been married 14 years." The dissolution of his marriage made him sad and destitute, but he had been able to find a position volunteering with the NGO, which provided some opportunities for per diems and workshop fees. His health improved once he got regular ARVs. He now felt he had a sense of purpose, because he was helping others (Informal discussion, PLHIV, Kitwe, May 19, 2011). Biomedicine, as well as his work with the NGO and other PLHIV, had transformed his life.

Sometimes these extraversion stories expressed gratitude to donors. One Zambian interviewee described his sickness and his family's financial destitution because of AIDS. He then was tested for HIV and started ARV medications. At that point in the interview, the man repeatedly and profusely thanked one of the authors for his medications, saying that ART had allowed him to return to work as a truck driver. He said, "My life is good. Now I can feed my family." Then, in a performance of positive living, he described how he took his medication daily, and when he was away from home, his wife called him to remind him about his drugs (Interview, PLHIV, Lusaka, March 2, 2011).

The three stories epitomized donors' desire for personal empowerment, since all three individuals had moved beyond their initial condition of illness, ostracism, and marginalization to become healthy, productive members of society. Such testimonies aligned with donors' desire to see results and with their faith in biomedicine and neoliberal responsibilization (Ferguson 2010). The telling of these stories became a way to gain continued opportunities, as seemed to be the case for the two PLHIV who worked with NGOs. The stories of gratitude to donors also helped to maintain positive relations with external actors who had the power to continue or curtail current benefits as well as bring future resources.

Finally, PLHIV *groups* utilized extraversion themes, building on the aforementioned individual approaches as well as claims of "authenticity." In the context of funding cuts in a projectified environment, groups needed to show that they were the "first" and most "in touch" with local PLHIV. They played to donors' desire to work with legitimate and representative community groups (Interview, FBO official, Lusaka, August 15, 2007; on NGOs, see Hilhorst 2003; Ellis 2011) For example, NZP+ groups often mentioned that they were the first PLHIV groups in any given neighborhood (FGDs, PLHIV groups, Livingstone, June 27, 2011 and Lusaka, March 23, 2011). They also claimed to "represent any PLHIV even if they are not a member of our organization or do not pay dues" (Interview, NZP+ official, Lusaka, August 17, 2007). In the context of the ZNAN scandal, NZP+ tried to capitalize on this authenticity, particularly since some PLHIV thought ZNAN had "used its privileged position with donors just to benefit itself" (Interview, PLHIV, Lusaka, March 22, 2011; see also Syed 2011). For some, ZNAN had never really represented PLHIV in the communities: "They don't know the life of the PLHIV" (Interview, PLHIV, Lusaka, March 30, 2011). Authenticity became a resource for extraversion with external actors.

Using Donor Practices in Extraversion: The Theme of Exclusion

In development interventions, donors set priorities and channel resources to "development insiders" in a process that serves to exacerbate differences with "development outsiders" (Boesten 2011). HIV exceptionalism has created new categories of development insiders and outsiders, new forms of exception and exclusion (Nguyen 2010, 177, 186, 209; see also Benton 2015; Patterson 2016). In our research, we noted exclusion around HIV status, geographic location, and broker position. In terms of HIV status, donors wanted to ensure they worked with PLHIV, and they often set criteria for project participation that only PLHIV (and sometimes, only particular PLHIV such as the very sick or children) could meet (Interview, NGO official, Lusaka, March 17, 2011). Because of the resources HIV could bring and despite the continued AIDS stigma, HIV had become popularly normalized and accepted as a "part of life." For example, a business woman considered how "now with HIV there is relief—with ARVs you cannot die within one year. So people prefer to get money that day because everyone will die, so there is no fear" (Interview, PLHIV, Zomba City, July 17, 2011). As a result, some people presented themselves as HIV positive to attract resources when they were not actually infected. The district coordinator for NAPHAM explained this situation in the context of registering new groups of PLHIV:

> False people come, but for someone to register their support group we ask them to take us to their group so we can come and meet these people. We meet them, if they are on ARVs we ask them [to] "show us your card" that shows where they were tested positive. We then know they want to join the group to benefit from NAPHAM's program. In each and every group we have met people falsifying their status. For example, 22 people came to register to say they were HIV positive and from a group, but those people admitted that they were just sent by a CBO chairman to attend. (Interview, NAPHAM coordinator, Zomba, June 28, 2011; see also Interview, NZP+ leader, Ndola, May 22, 2011)

We researchers were not immune from similar incidents. During our field-work, some HIV-negative people presented themselves as HIV positive in hopes of receiving some benefit. In one case, two entire villages came to meet one author because her local contact had misinformed the village head that she was from an NGO. Unusual in support groups, many men attended the meeting and were especially keen to provide their testimonies and present themselves as being gender aware (Participant observations and FGDs, Lusaka, Kitwe, Ndola, Lilongwe, Zomba, Karonga, February–September 2011). In these examples, dependent agents play up what many donors view to be both a weakness and an essential criteria for assistance—a positive HIV status—to get resources.

Geographic location was another donor-related theme. Donor resources tend to be concentrated in areas where they can maximize returns such as in accessible communities and communities where many organizations already work (FGDs and participant observations, Malawi and Zambia, February–September 2011; see also Chinsinga 2007, 92). For example, one support group in Karonga Boma that was situated close to Karonga center received a farm, fertilizer, seeds, goats, porridge, and trainings on nutrition (FGD, PLHIV group, Karonga Boma, Karonga, August 20, 2011). Other groups situated in major urban centers along the main Chilumba Road to Tanzania reported that they received farms, farm inputs, and training sessions from several NGOs (FGDs, PLHIV groups, Kasowa, Karonga, August 22, 2011; Puse, Karonga, August 23, 2011; Lupembe, Karonga, August 26, 2011). And several Lusaka PLHIV groups were approached by NGOs and FBOs, even if they had had failed projects in the past (Fgds, PLHIV groups, Lusaka, April 7, 2011 and March 23, 2011).

In contrast, some rural groups received little assistance. Both NAPHAM and NZP+ district coordinators recognized this problem, but they also lacked vehicles or funds for fuel to help these groups (Interview, NZP+ leader, Kabwe, April 18, 2011; Participant observation, NAPHAM executive meeting, Karonga Boma, August 19, 2011). In Malawi, members of one support group in Nbande that was situated 12 km from Karonga along the Chipita Road said that "NAPHAM is biased in selecting groups to be assisted." Another member said "other groups receive loans, sugar, cooking oil, soap, and salt—and here nothing at all." A third added, "They choose groups that are close to town but not as far as here" (FGD, Karonga, August 25, 2011). A Zambian group located 14 km from Livingstone asserted, "Lack of transportation means we just hear about these projects but [there's] nothing in this location; we are getting nothing from these Global Funds. There is no NGO to support us" (FGD, PLHIV group, Livingstone, June 27, 2011). And the original NAPHAM group in Karonga district (it was based in Chilumba) said it became overlooked when the NAPHAM office moved to the urban area of Karonga Boma (FGD, PLHIV group, Chilumba, Karonga, September 3, 2011).

The theme of rural exclusion was even used by groups that had received donor support. The abovementioned Nbande group, for example, had gotten farming support, money for goats, soap, mosquito nets, and trainings from NGOs, but it continued to play up its isolation (FGD, PLHIV group, Karonga August 25, 2011). Similarly, one group located 18 km from Livingstone had received donor funding to raise goats and pigs. The project was very successful, but the group complained extensively about "being left out" (FDG, PLHIV group, Livingstone, June 27, 2011). And despite being targeted with farming inputs, trainings, and medical supplies, the Fulirwa group said that it had not received material support from NAPHAM for a long time (FGD, PLHIV group, Karonga September 2, 2011)

Complaints about exclusion could also target brokers, who were essential to help groups gain benefits but were also uniquely situated to utilize those benefits. While most groups recognized that they needed brokers, some asserted that brokers were selective in how they channeled benefits, favoring the brokers' relatives, friends, home regions, or coreligionists

(FGD, PLHIV group, Fulirwa, Karonga, September 2, 2011). One support group in Chilumba suggested that the NAPHAM district coordinator's favoritism toward her own area meant that "when there are good things like trainings, we are not involved" (Fgds, PLHIV group, Chilumba Galizon, Karonga, September 1, 2011; see participant observation, NAPHAM executive meeting, Karonga Boma, August 19, 2011). Another group became suspicious when they compared themselves to other organizations: "We are just hearing that our friends have received loans and goats, but here nothing despite giving them reports" (FGD, PLHIV group, Mwenitete, Karonga, August 24, 2011). After the ZNAN scandal in Zambia, CBOs feared that CHAZ (which had taken over ZNAN's grants) would ignore them because it preferred church PLHIV groups and HBC programs. One PLHIV said, "ZNAN was for the community groups; CHAZ is for the churches. We have no one for us now" (FGD, PLHIV group, Lusaka, March 30, 2011). In a few groups, members extended the exclusion theme to claim that leaders had stolen group funds, leaving everyone else penniless (Participant observation, NAPHAM executive meeting, Karonga Boma, August 19, 2011; Fgds, PLHIV groups, Lusaka, April 14, 2011 and March 24, 2011). Being "left out" became a theme expressed to donors and researchers; exclusion was both a reality and a tool for gaining possible resources.

These allegations of favoritism must be interpreted in a context in which brokers must maintain ties to kith and kin because of their precarious position. They may use the benefits that come from being a broker (e.g., high pay and access to resources, per diems, and travel allowances) when they have the opportunity to do so, because these benefits will not last forever. Employment contracts tend to be short-term and donor projects end. Yet these behaviors opened the door for the local PLHIV whom these brokers linked to donors to engage in extraversion around themes of nepotism and favoritism. Such themes may resonate with donors' views of the continent and lead donors who espouse efficiency and equality to rethink projects and their relations with brokers (Krause 2014). We return to the impact of extraversion on donors' policies and programs in the next chapter.

Extraversion for Training and by Training

While extraversion could be used as a tool to get many types of resources, a common resource that groups sought was training, because of its aforementioned benefits. This desired objective fit well with donors' concerns about fostering a sustainable AIDS response (see Chapter 2), since groups needed the skills to apply for money, run projects, and report results (FGDs, PLHIV group, Lusaka, March 30, 2011 and April 1, 2011). PLHIV groups argued that their very lack of capacity—their weaknesses —justified their inclusion in trainings where report writing, data collection, project management, and budget making were taught (Interview, FBO official, Lusaka, March 31, 2011). The call for training also tapped into Western stereotypes of African institutions that emphasize poor management and inefficiencies (Ellis 2011).

In the following example of extraversion, one Malawian group leader highlighted his group's problems in order to lobby for future training opportunities:

> We have complaints: lack of love from family members; these people are orphans and widows; others are not working, have no business. We consulted NAPHAM and City Assembly to help us; we fill forms but up to now to no avail. In 2006 we filled a MARDEF loan form but up to now, nothing is happening. This group comprises of different congregations but we are sick and to travel is not easy—so we need bicycles. Food is a very big problem; we are taking ARVs without food. A lot of people have been sick for a very long time, hence all their funds have been consumed and they have children and it is difficult to pay their school fees. We are over working and hence our immunity is deteriorating fast. Lots of them are breadwinners and to get loans is not easy because they say you are about to die. We need farm inputs [i.e., fertilizer subsidy]. We are side-lined. (Participant observation, PLHIV group meeting, Zomba City, Zomba, July 13, 2011)

All of these problems connected directly to the next series of planned NAPHAM trainings on youth and child therapy, financial management, and livelihoods (including farming). Although group members had previously been included in trainings, the leader said they were "side-lined." He then pointed out the group's current activities and the lessons the group had learned at previous NAPHAM trainings to make the case for why it should receive continuous support. While we do not deny the problems the group faced, one goal of the leader's performance was to highlight these problems in a pitch for trainings.

Trainings are not only important as a source of resources, but they also become the arena in which PLHIV learn to perfect extraversion themes.

For example, at one MANET+ training in Mponela, Malawi, the facilitator started by asking, "How can you facilitate community mobilization programs when you cannot talk about yourself?" He then gave his testimony before asking the participants to provide theirs (Participant observation, Training session, June 26, 2011). Similarly, an NGO that supports women in Karonga "tell[s] us [the group members] to declare our status to the community to motivate them" (FGD, PLHIV group, Karonga Boma, Karonga, August 20, 2011). It was apparent that PLHIV had learned these lessons, for during the FGDs they often told their personal stories of contracting HIV or living with AIDS even in response to general questions about HIV. As indicated above, sometimes these responses could be gendered, though not always. In a Malawi group, one man explained, for example, that he contracted HIV through "drinking beer (hence I lost my memory) and sleeping without condoms." Then another woman stood up and revealed that "I'm HIV positive because of revenge: I discovered my husband was having affairs, so I decided to do the same. Now I am the one who is HIV positive" (Participant observation, PLHIV group, Nsondole, Zomba, July 6, 2011). Members of one Zambian group emphasized the depression and suicidal thoughts they experienced after discovering their HIV status. While we do not doubt their stories of anguish, it was notable that all six of seven group members used the terms depression, suicide, and psychosocial support—themes highlighted in trainings (FGD, PLHIV group, Lusaka, March 23, 2011). Trainings became a resource, as well as an arena in which to perfect extraversion language.

In this section we have highlighted how PLHIV may use extraversion on themes of the diseased body, the marginalized PLHIV, the entrepreneurial woman, and the healthy, empowered PLHIV. Collectively, groups may stress their "founder status" to increase their authenticity and legitimacy. As a mode of action, extraversion is fluid and dynamic, with particular themes stressed at different times and for different audiences. For example, groups may emphasize work with AIDS orphans when they speak with FBOs, since FBOs often assist children (Interview, FBO official, Lusaka, August 15, 2007). Because donors cannot serve all PLHIV, dependent agents may use donors' own priorities and programs to cry "exclusion" as a means to gain resources. Trainings may become the objective of many extraversion attempts and ultimately, an important arena in which extraversion is learned.

RESISTANCE BELOW THE LINE

While not public and direct, resistance below the line was evident in the use of euphemisms, foot-dragging, stretching the rules, and reframing the issue. These efforts seek to "thwart surveillance," and thus, they often are not interpreted as resistance by the powerful. But resistance below the line is "real politics" because these actions have the potential to affect the activities of the dominant player (see Scott 1990, 200). By using this resistance, dependent agents recognize that they need to "play the game" to appease external actors even if they fundamentally oppose the assumptions that underlie the game. While hidden transcripts may not bring resistance directly into the public realm (for doing so may be dangerous), they do provide an alternative vision, a way of practicing autonomy; they are illustrative of the fact that no dependent agent is "entirely submissive or entirely insubordinate" (Scott 1990, 192).

With euphemisms, the dependent agent "disguises the message just enough to skirt retaliation.... The veiling of the message represents the application of varnish" (Scott 1990, 152). The use of indirect talk was most evident in discussion of one's HIV status, and its practice illustrates how not all dependent agents engage the AIDS official story's demand for public disclosure of one's HIV status. We illustrated above that some PLHIV explicitly talked about their HIV infection, using extraversion to echo Western assumptions about individual responsibility in sexual behavior and gender inequalities (see Anderson 2015). Yet not all PLHIV wanted to make their HIV infection stories available for public discussion, for reasons of privacy, personal reputation, and family pressure (see Nguyen 2010). Instead, they spoke in euphemisms that showed just enough individual responsibility to fit within donors' neoliberal focus on individual accountability and PLHIV responsibilization and also enough secrecy to protect themselves. One man explained that now he "had turned from a past life," without explaining what that past life was (Interview, PLHIV, Lusaka, May 9, 2011). Another woman simply said, "There were some bad actions in my past" (FGD, PLHIV group, Lusaka, March 22, 2011).

Foot-dragging related to donors' requirements for projects such as report writing. In Zambia, several HBC groups were notoriously late in submitting their reports on the number of PLHIV and AIDS orphans they served. But report writing was time consuming and challenging, particularly for caregivers with limited education. Caregivers wanted to serve others, not fill out forms (FGD, caregiver group, Kitwe, May 19, 2011;

Interview, FBO official, Lusaka, April 8, 2011). Yet groups also realized that they had to complete forms to continue to get resources. Foot-dragging was subversive, and brokers spent a lot of time "nagging" local groups to complete their reports (Informal conversation, FBO volunteer, Lusaka, April 9, 2011; Participant observation, NAPHAM executive meeting, Karonga Boma, August 19, 2011).

The influx of AIDS resources contributed to the rise of professional aid recipients, but some of those recipients "stretched the rules" to increase their benefits. Stretching the rules enabled dependent agents to gain resources while minimizing compliance with official policies. An NGO director in Malawi explained how the NGO pays its staff members USD 100 per day for expenses for work-related travel, making travel very profitable. Yet, the NGO experienced problems with people claiming more days for expenses than they were actually traveling (Informal discussion, NGO director, Zomba, July 25, 2011). In both countries, NGO officials mentioned incidents when NGO workers or volunteers falsified travel claims to maximize the money they received for attending meetings and trainings. Similarly, the representatives of PLHIV groups received an allowance to cover transport, accommodation, lunch, and refreshments at trainings, but sometimes attendees tried to claim fuel costs with receipts that had been "adjusted" (Informal discussions, NGO representatives, Lilongwe, Lusaka, Zomba and Karonga, June–September 2011). Given the large fluctuations in fuel costs during 2011, these adjustments were not initially suspected. These examples show how individuals can submit to the system's rules—attending trainings, submitting receipts—while also using the ambiguities in the system to benefit themselves.

Stretching the rules was also evident in training attendance. While donors and participants valued trainings, trainings had an opportunity cost for attendees: trainings might involve travel and substantial time away from home, family obligations, and/or a business. If trainings were held in the home community, other demands (like childcare, cooking, and housework) could pull at participants' time, particularly if those trainees were women. As a result, sometimes people did not attend trainings (FGD, PLHIV group, Karonga Boma, Karonga, August 20, 2011). At other times, they attended but only came for part of the training. One HBC group leader complained that "people come late and leave early," noting that these stragglers often managed to make training sessions in time for morning tea and lunch (Informal conversation, Kitwe, May 19, 2011). This behavior enabled dependent agents to do "just enough" to reaffirm the system's validity and to gain benefits, while not allowing the system to control their autonomous agenda. Such actions did not require that participants abandon obligations to kith and kin, the social structures that would bring security and assistance if (or when) donors were gone. Furthermore, given the fact that, as indicated above, dependent agents saw limited value in trainings, "just enough" attendance to subversively reaffirm donors' objectives was logical.

Additionally, resistance was evident when PLHIV sought to redefine the issue, often using the language or concerns of donors to lobby for additional or different policies. In the process, they subversively sought to change the official AIDS story. Brokers were crucial participants in these processes, for they best knew the language, ideals, and policies of donors. For example, as Chapter 2 showed, many PLHIV groups had come to expect food distribution (Interview, church AIDS coordinator, Lusaka, February 25, 2011), and the vast majority reported that "access to food" was their biggest concern. Brokers sometimes encouraged these complaints. For example, when one Malawian woman criticized NAPHAM because "in the past a long time ago they were giving us food but now counselling only," the complaint led to an enthusiastic discussion that the discussion facilitator jovially encouraged. His laughter led another woman to say, "Can someone get full with counselling?" and a third to confirm that "it is not effective" (FGD, PLHIV group, Kasowa, Karonga, August 22, 2011).

Even though brokers urged these criticisms, donor officials often dismissed these complaints, with one in Zambia asserting that such statements were found "everywhere you go" (Interview, NGO official, Kitwe, May 20, 2011). In response to donors' unwillingness to engage their criticisms, many groups tried to redefine the issue of food distribution not as "a handout" but as an essential component of local "capacity building." They used crucial jargon that fit with donors' themes of responsibilization and sustainability. Without food, they argued, PLHIV could not take their medication; nonadherence made it difficult to reach donors' goal of successful treatment projects. They also argued that without food, PLHIV had no physical energy for income-generating projects (FGDs, PLHIV groups, Lusaka, March 2, 2011; February 25, 2011 and May 9, 2011; FGDs, PLHIV groups, Karonga, August–September, 2011). Low PLHIV participation would undermine donors' goal of income-generating projects that fostered a sustainable AIDS response.

Some groups sought to redefine HIV vulnerability in hopes of shaping the AIDS response. In one case, several church groups wanted to include HIV-negative people in their AIDS programs, stressing that everyone in poverty is vulnerable to HIV, and thus, everyone should have access to income-generating projects and trainings. One broker (who was a pastor) said, "It is not our sero-status but our poverty that draws us together" (FGDs, caregiver and PLHIV groups, Ndola, May 22, 2011). This pastor had connections to FBOs and some Western congregations, who depended on him to lead his local congregants in the AIDS response. As an intermediary, he was able to combine his parishioners' desire to access resources with donors' desire to help the poorest members in society in order to redefine the issue away from AIDS (and potentially, the sexual behavior that facilitates HIV transmission) to poverty (Interview, FBO official, Ndola, May 22, 2011; see Krakauer and Newbery 2007).

While the actions highlighted here are not revolutionary, as Chapter 4 shows, they still may affect donor objectives, processes, and programs. Scott (1990) writes that it is at the intersection of public politics, with its explicit rhetoric and structures of power and domination, and private actions that never slip into the public space, where subversion is possible. We do not claim that all dependent agents utilize these acts of resistance below the line, for their use requires an opportunity to do so. For example, stretching the rules on training attendance may only be possible for those with a plausible excuse (e.g., a sick child who needs tending). Additionally, we recognize that even subversive resistance requires courage: not everyone is bold enough to turn in reports late, show up for trainings just before lunch, or rewrite a receipt. These factors mean the strategy is fluidly employed, illustrating even further the ability of dependent agents to respond to particular contexts and to act in creative ways.

Conclusion

This chapter has explored three strategies of dependent agents: performances of compliance, extraversion, and resistance below the line. These dynamic strategies incorporate technologies of jargon such as "positive living" and "activism," as well as donor-promoted structures such as group rules and report writing. In performances of compliance, many of our dependent agents dressed the part and engaged the actions expected of them, such as clapping for donor projects, memorizing information, dancing, and in what is a simple but important form of compliance, merely showing up at donor events. Many also used specific extraversion narratives and images such as the diseased body, the marginalized PLHIV, or the empowered PLHIV. Brokers often helped groups to perfect extraversion and performances of compliance, though they could sometimes become the target of extraversion strategies related to exclusion. Resistance below the line allowed dependent agents to simultaneously benefit from and challenge the dominant AIDS narrative.

We have shown that these strategies are dynamic and unevenly adopted: some groups and individual PLHIV have learned to perform for donors, while others have not. This dynamism was evident in our fieldwork: as groups and individuals got to know us, they may have realized that their performances had little leverage with us and thus, they jettisoned them.

Finally, our fieldwork raises a crucial point about trainings, or the venue in which performances of compliance are learned and the rhetoric of extraversion is acquired. They are where people learn to play the game. We discovered that trainings play an even larger role in the continuance of the AIDS enterprise than what Watkins and Swidler (2013) assert (see also Smith 2003). While they provide material benefits and help donors train people for a "sustainable" AIDS response, they also teach people how to continue to ask for benefits (including trainings) in ways that both affirm donors' goals (through the performances of compliance) and play to external actors' sympathies and assumptions about PLHIV in Africa (through extraversion).

NOTES

1. *Nsima/Nshima* is the staple food in Malawi and Zambia, made from maize flour.
2. *Chiponde* is a nutritious porridge.
3. *Fisi* is a cultural practice that occurs in southern Malawi whereby a woman engages in extramarital sex with another member of the family, a friend of the husband, a traditional practitioner, or a hired man known as the *"fisi"* (hyena) to increase the likelihood that she conceives (See Anderson 2015, 138–139, 2012, 272–273).

Complex Power on the Margins:
The Implications of Dependent Agency

Abstract The implications of dependent agency are multifaceted. First, it may influence donors' ability to achieve their objectives, while also reinforcing the status quo and undermining local solidarity. Second, it may shape democratization by challenging liberal citizenship and undermining transparency and accountability in decision-making. Despite these limitations, dependent agency also illustrates local people's desire for participation and their nascent demands for the powerful to be held accountable. The work concludes by exploring how the concept of dependent agency may shape scholarship on African politics, international relations, and global health.

Keywords Implications of dependent agency · Donor objectives · Local solidarity · Democratization · Global health

Dominated people have always used behind-the-scenes activities to subvert the actions and structures of the powerful. During the dictatorship of Idi Amin in Uganda (1971–1979), rural farmers quietly uprooted their coffee trees to plant food crops in order to survive, an action that undermined a regime reliant on coffee exports for revenue (Bunker 1987; see Hyden 1980 on Tanzania). In *The Emperor's New Clothes*, villagers compliment the emperor's new wardrobe, which in reality is no clothing at all. Ironically, when the king parades his nakedness publicly, it is the most

© The Author(s) 2017
E.-L. Anderson, A.S. Patterson, *Dependent Agency in the Global Health Regime*, DOI 10.1057/978-1-137-58148-8_4

powerless member of society—a child—who points out his foolishness. But it is too late: for the villagers' performances of compliance have subverted the king's authority (Andersen 1837). In his 1989 song "Beasts of No Nation," the late Fela Kuti challenges the production and reproduction of structures and ideologies of domination under military rule in Nigeria (Hungbo 2014, 167). A Senegalese woman in a polygamous relationship manipulates her husband's sexual desires to get him to pay the school fees for her child (Informal discussion, rural Senegalese woman, Ndoulo, May 5, 1995). Our work has extended our knowledge of such subversive activities into the context of donor AIDS projects in Africa.

This book has developed the concept of *dependent agency*. In Chapter 1, we defined dependent agency as the condition in which actors can simultaneously act and be dependent. We explained how donor competition, foreign aid uncertainty, development discourses that promote grassroots participation, norms that define health as a human right, and the rise of the AIDS enterprise created opportunities for dependent agency. In Chapter 2, we showed that dependent agency is situated in particular contexts through an examination of the cases of Malawi and Zambia. We argued that although these two countries are extremely dependent on donor funding and face acute poverty—they have tight corners for agentic behavior—their citizens were not without agency. Changing economic fortunes and donor priorities presented new spaces into which dependent agents might enter and new issues around which they might act. Chapter 3 then interrogated the nuances of specific strategies that dependent agents utilize. Drawing upon our empirical data and extending from the work of James C. Scott and Jean-François Bayart, we highlighted three: performances of compliance, extraversion, and resistance below the line. *Performances of compliance* included echoing the official story and holding powerful actors accountable through charges of hypocrisy, while *extraversion* entailed a variety of PLHIV testimonies and claims of donor exclusion. Donor-funded trainings were often the site for learning extraversion motifs and perfecting performances of compliance. *Resistance below the line* included the use of euphemisms, stretching the rules, and foot dragging. All three strategies embodied everyday actions that are "subtle, indirect and non-confrontational"; and through them, our dependent agents showed "persistence, prudence and individual effort to accomplish a specific goal" (Thomson 2014, 111). These goals included obtaining material benefits (no matter how small) and volunteer and/or paid positions, as well as increasing one's social status. A desire for personal enrichment rooted in social pressures and familial obligations led dependent agents to seek such benefits.

In this concluding chapter, we investigate the implications of these small agentic acts for socioeconomic development, democratization, and the study of Africa in international politics. We question how dependent agency shapes donors' ability to achieve their objectives. Patrick Chabal (2014, xvi) asserts that local agency has the potential to undermine power relations between the powerful and the marginalized (in our case, between donors and local aid recipients) and to lead to public forms of resistance (see Scott 1990). While we found this effect in a few cases, we demonstrate that it was more common that dependent agency reinforced the status quo and undermined grassroots solidarity. In terms of democratization, we argue that dependent agency may challenge the formation of liberal citizens who hold the state accountable, and dependent agents' strategies may undermine the transparency and accountability needed for democracy. Yet through their private actions these dependent actors show both a desire to express themselves and a nascent demand for the powerful to be accountable. We conclude by exploring how dependent agency may shape theories of African agency within the fields of international relations and global health politics.

Dependent Agency and Development

While the actions of dependent agents seem solely focused on getting short-term benefits like food or per diems, these activities also may shape the very development processes that dependent agents rely on. Donors may go along with performances of compliance, since such performances can bolster donors' own arguments for funding and/or program expansion. They may ignore or downplay extraversion, though donors may react if extraversion questions their *raison d'etre* and legitimacy. Donors are more likely to respond to resistance below the line than the other two strategies, because it directly impacts the efficiency of programs. We then demonstrate how dependent agency may affect the ties of trust and solidarity that scholars assert are needed to foster socioeconomic development and democracy (see Putnam 1994; Coleman 1988). The drive to perform, extravert, and resist may divide community members, particularly since only some individuals succeed in these efforts. Finally, we show that dependent agency fits within a neoliberal discourse that values rationality, responsibility, and initiative, but also damages community empowerment and sustainable development.

Reacting to the Strategies

The majority of donor officials we encountered were aware of the complex nuances of local agency which shape their program efforts. Off the record, they critically reflected on the impact that agency has on their operations and the effectiveness of their programs. Many recognized that dependent agents engaged in performances of compliance, including praising donor projects, answering HIV-related questions in the "right way," and displaying positive health behaviors. Sometimes these performances undermined the donor's objectives, particularly if there was a discrepancy between the public and hidden transcripts. For example, one donor official reported that the information local translators presented did not align with what the official witnessed during monitoring and evaluation visits in communities (Informal discussion, donor official, Lilongwe, June 29, 2014). This discrepancy made monitoring projects difficult.

As patrons who were the audience for the performers, donors had a role to play: they were expected to praise the performers. But donors were not merely altruistic. Performances could benefit donors because they generated anecdotes of success that could be included in final reports and funding pleas (see, e.g., Population Council 2010). One PLHIV group meeting at a donor-funded AIDS clinic in Lusaka illustrated this dynamic. At the start of the meeting, a donor-paid community organizer peppered members with questions about HIV: "What is a CD4 count?"[1] "What foods should you eat to stay healthy?" "How do we prevent HIV infection?" Group members answered dutifully. After the meeting, the donor official who had attended the meeting proudly said, "See how these support groups teach so much information? The knowledge of AIDS is so high" (Participant observation, AIDS clinic, Lusaka, May 5, 2011). While it was apparent that the members knew much about AIDS because of their involvement with the group, they did not always act on this knowledge. During the FGD that followed the meeting, some participants reported that PLHIV sometimes do not use condoms to prevent HIV transmission (FDG, PLHIV group, Lusaka, May 5, 2011). Regardless, the group's performance of its knowledge enabled the donor official to claim a "success" in terms of its HIV education programs.

In a broader sense, donors' acquiescence to the performances promoted the status quo. Even though donors recognized the "allowance culture," performances that mimicked donors' rhetoric, and the creation of "professional aid recipients," they did not typically speak of these behaviors in public forums or criticize the individuals who engaged in them. When they did, they couched their comments in phrases like "I know we don't talk about it but" (Participant observations, public forums with HIV stakeholders, Lilongwe, June–July 2014; Informal discussions, donor officials, Lilongwe, June–July 2014; Lusaka, August 2007 and March–May 2011). When they accepted performances, they acquiesced to local power structures that enabled some actors to repeatedly access training opportunities or NGO benefits to the exclusion of others. When they praised the ability of clinic attendees to explain positive health behaviors, they did not question how structures of poverty or gender inequality might prevent PLHIV from embracing such behaviors (see Anderson 2015). Performances of compliance enabled donors to avoid the structural obstacles to development; in the process, donors perpetuated what James Ferguson (1994) terms the "anti-politics machine."

In terms of extraversion, donors' reactions were colored by the ways that dependent agents framed their claims. Donors often demonstrated empathy when agents spoke of their poverty, hunger, health problems, and exclusion from programs, though they often did not promise assistance. For example, one FBO official in Zambia listened to and sympathized with a local PLHIV, but in the end, only offered, "I will pray to the Lord Almighty that he will deliver you from these problems. God can do it" (Participant observation, PLHIV group, Ndola, June 9, 2014). A few donor officials became irate with extraversion efforts, as the following quote during an FGD in Zambia indicates. The PLHIV group had been asked about its challenges and successes. As was typical during FGDs, members reported many challenges, a pattern that indicated how extraversion was commonplace. But when group members were silent when asked about the group's accomplishments and strengths, the donor official responded:

Don't just talk about what you don't have and what you want. Look inside yourself, your group...You just want to answer the question by talking about your challenges, but she wants to know the good things. Like the business training, the loans you got. And before you even talk about the loans, talk about the skills you learned. The people you worked for. The businesses you started. (FDG, PLHIV group, Kabwe, April 18, 2011)

This public challenge to extraversion was a relative anomaly. It was more common for donors to engage in a delicate back-and-forth with dependent agents over control of the narrative. Dependent agents outlined their problems; donors empathized and sometimes, when they perceived their legitimacy was at stake, they responded materially. For example, some church-based caregiving groups framed their demands for material benefits in light of ideals of Christian compassion. Not to be outdone on religious rhetoric, FBO officials then spoke about how religious beliefs undergird their projects. Sometimes they felt they needed to provide groups with material benefits in order to illustrate their religious sincerity. One respondent said, "We know that 99 percent of the people who are providing care are doing so because they follow Jesus and 'love their neighbors as themselves'. And as followers of Christ, we [the international FBO] feel we must help them. So when they say they need gloves to work, we try to get that for them. Or if they ask for bicycles, we have tried to provide" (Interview, FBO official, Lusaka, August 15, 2007). Extraversion that stressed religious faith brought benefits because these themes cut to the FBO's core mission.

When dependent agents used resistance below the line, donors were more likely to react since these activities could undermine project efficiency. As indicated in Chapter 3, stretching the rules included "creative accounting" or misreporting workshop attendance in order to divert resources for private gain. In response, donors changed how they dispersed AIDS monies to government agencies and NGOs. In Malawi, the publication of the Global Fund audit that revealed corruption of donor funds was followed by an audit of donor funds to government, which revealed that an estimated MWK 13 billion (USD 30 million) was not accounted for over a 6-month period (OIG 2012). One program manager at a major donor organization pointed to systematic failures and explained that "Cashgate [as the scandal was called] was the final nail following the decline in faith in governance" (Interview, donor official, Lilongwe, June 26, 2014). This statement indicates that donors had previously been aware of the small ways in which dependent agents had stretched the rules for allowable program spending and financial accounting reports. In both countries, major donors also placed technical advisors within the government to act as their "eyes on the ground" to oversee funding. Because the payment of travel and per diem allowances had become a particular concern, these technical advisors were responsible for signing off on payments and verifying the details of local-level training activities (Interviews, donor officials, Lilongwe, June–July 2014; donor official, Lusaka, February 23, 2011). One respondent explained the reason for this change in policies:

> Previously we [the donor] could have six people, their names appearing [on the attendance records for] . . . various activities happening at the same time and you wonder how they could have been in all those places at the same time. So that is not able to happen right now because every little training, we [the technical advisors] have to be [present] in it. It is purely like the private sector: we want every coin to be able to be accounted for. (Interview, donor technical advisor, Lilongwe, July 27, 2014)

The speaker indicates both how dependent agents had sought to maneuver around the rules and the pressure for the AIDS enterprise to transparently account for "every coin."

Over the years of our fieldwork, we noted changes in donors' operating procedures. In response to foot dragging on report writing, in Zambia some donors made reports due less frequently and simplified forms (Interview, FBO official, Lusaka, March 30, 2011). For reimbursement for trainings, donors developed stricter rules on allowances and attendance at workshops. In response to fuel claims that were suspicious, some training organizations imposed a cap on how much they would pay for travel allowances (Participant observations and informal discussions, training sessions with PLHIV, Malawi, June–September 2011).

Patrick Chabal (2014, xvi) writes that agency is not "a mere re-action" or "reflex opposition." Instead, it "seeks to oppose or undermine the constraining pressure, which restricts the ability of ordinary people to live, function, work or play as they see fit." Performances, extraversion, and resistance below the line had the potential to undermine the power and legitimacy of dominant actors and provide greater degrees of freedom for local individuals. In theory, if donors were not careful about how they responded to these strategies, they could find local people questioning their motives or turning from their efforts. While relatively uncommon, this outcome did occur in a few cases. One Zambian PLHIV explained that many NGOs had come to his neighborhood to work on AIDS. But because these groups did not respond when local people explained their needs (through extraversion), people became suspicious and started to believe that donors promised but rarely delivered (Interview, PLHIV, Lusaka, March 1, 2011). In other communities, some PLHIV reported that they "hang back" to see if the NGO is really serious before they invest energy or time in a project (FGD, PLHIV group, Ndola, May 23, 2011; Interview, PLHIV, Makunganya, Zomba, July 29, 2011). Thus, when donors do not pay attention to the under-the-radar strategies of the dominated, they may find that their broader project objectives are undermined by suspicion and low participation.

Undermining Trust and Solidarity

Strategies of dependent agency may also shape local solidarity (e.g., a sense of unity around shared objectives) and trust (e.g., confidence that others will do what they promise). Robert Putnam (1994) asserts that such values are crucial for economic development and democratic deepening because they enable groups to overcome the free rider problem by predicting the behavior of their members. Francis Fukuyama (1995, 27) writes specifically about trust: "If people ... trust one another because they are all operating according to a common set of ethical norms, doing business costs less. Such a society will be better able to innovate organizationally, since the high degree of trust will permit a wide variety of social relationships to emerge" (see also Warren 1999). In the vast majority of PLHIV and caregiving groups we encountered there was a strong sense of trust and solidarity. PLHIV in almost every group said they were "brothers and sisters," "one family," and "of one mind and heart" (FGDs, PLHIV and caregiver groups, Lusaka, Ndola, Kabwe, Mumbwa, Livingstone, Kitwe, Zomba, and Karonga, February–September 2011). They also reported a strong sense of obligation to others, because "someone helped me in the past when I was ill or had nothing to eat, so when I see a need and can help, I need to return the favor" (FGD, caregiver group, Kitwe, May 20, 2011). They also wanted to protect others from HIV: "I have knowledge about HIV and I must share my knowledge with my community" (FGD, PLHIV group, Lusaka, March 22, 2011).

Yet, as Chapter 3 showed, because AIDS resources were limited and because donors channelled these resources in unequal ways (Boesten 2011; Nguyen 2010; Benton 2015), individuals sought to portray themselves as worthy recipients. Even though PLHIV have multiple identities (e.g., family member, community participant, religious believer, PLHIV, gendered person), extraversion necessitated that they craft their identity to align with donors' priorities. In the process, they could exclude impoverished friends and neighbors (see Patterson 2015). The resulting inequalities could undermine solidarity, as the following story told by the leader of a PLHIV group illustrates:

We were both HIV-positive and HIV-negative people when we started [our group] in 2000. The HIV-negative would care for the positive. This was before ART so care was central. In 2008 we decided to affiliate with NZP+ and that meant all the HIV-negative people had to leave. The [NZP+] constitution says that it is only for HIV-positive people. The people who were negative didn't believe this; they even called in the [NZP+] district coordinator to explain the policy. So the negative people weren't happy when they had to leave; they took part of the group's money and over half of the members. (FGD, PLHIV group, Ndola, May 23, 2011)

Because PLHIV identity mattered to the donors who supported NZP+, people emphasized this identity. People who had previously worked together became divided: some HIV-negative people felt hurt and angry because they had devoted themselves to care for PLHIV; some PLHIV suspected that the HIV-negative people just wanted donor benefits and did not really care about their HIV-positive neighbors. The PLHIV group then faced challenges because of lost members and funds (Informal discussion, NZP+ leader, Ndola, May 23, 2011).

In other communities, similar divisions existed between PLHIV groups and CBOs, HBC groups, and FBOs. One Malawian PLHIV group reported that it was "having problems to work [sic] with their CBO, [and so] now we will work alone." Other Malawian PLHIV groups perceived that CBOs dominated decision-making around AIDS resources (Participant observation, NAPHAM executive meeting, Karonga, August 19, 2011). In some Zambian churches, PLHIV groups were suspicious of caregiving groups, asserting that "they always get all of the benefits" when donors come (FGD, PLHIV group, Lusaka, March 9, 2011). In all of these cases, donors' willingness to reward the groups or individuals that used testimonies that aligned with donors' AIDS discourses pitted poor people against one another for resources. In the process, solidarity was eroded. Since solidarity is a crucial asset that poor people have to foster their own development and to increase their political voice, this loss further marginalized them (Branch and Mampilly 2015). One PLHIV group leader reaffirmed this point: "If we continue to insist that PLHIV have their own groups, we are just perpetuating the stigma on AIDS...We will then just keep fighting and that helps no one" (Interview, PLHIV, Mpika, July 4, 2011).

Finally, as can occur in civil society groups (Patterson 2003), PLHIV organizations may suffer from internal distrust, particularly with respect to control of monetary resources, which is the most hoped-for outcome of dependent agency strategies. One NZP+ officer explained: "In the past, there have been groups where one leader just takes the money that the group might get for a project, and this then leads to mistrust in the group and loss of morale" (Interview, Lusaka, March 9, 2011). A PLHIV echoed this point: "Money issues can really divide people and erode trust in a group" (Interview, Kabwe, April 18, 2011), while the leader of a church-based PLHIV group said, "[Members trust] each other, but as you know, where there are people... We are all sinners. There can be someone who is not good" (Interview, PLHIV, Lusaka, February 24, 2011). As we've shown, dependent agency may give some people access to resources because they effectively utilize extraversion or performances of compliance. This unequal access can fuel distrust. The link between dependent agency and intragroup trust merits further investigation.

Shaping the Broader Development Agenda

The prevailing development orthodoxy has emphasized sustainability of projects by fostering rational, agentic, and responsibilized citizens who can develop their own communities without a long-term commitment of donor aid. In theory, if local people are trained and given inputs, they then can continue projects indefinitely and independently. This neoliberal approach also assumes that if some community members benefit through development processes, the community as a whole will gain (Scherz 2014; Harvey 2005; Ferguson 2010, 172). The dependent agents we studied embodied many attributes that neoliberalism values: they took the initiative, rationally acted on their interests, and illustrated a sense of responsibility to family (though not necessarily to the community). Yet they also challenged this neoliberal discourse in three crucial ways.

First, because dependent agents faced pressure to provide for family, their use of extraversion, resistance below the line, and performances of compliance does not necessarily promote the *community*'s socioeconomic advancement. For example, one PLHIV group in Zambia told the story of money it received for an income-generating project:

[Our project] was supposed to be a revolving fund. A few [members] who got the loans would then start a business and then repay; then the next would get a loan... Those leaders who first got [the loans] said it was a small amount and they could not really make a business. So they just declined to pay back so that we would all benefit ... Even though they signed a form saying they'd pay back, we haven't seen anything. (FGD, PLHIV group. Lusaka, April 7, 2011)

Another group member then explained why the leaders thought they could keep the money: "They said that since it was meant for the [HIV] infected people and they were infected, they refused to return the money. They said it was for their own use; they were entitled to it" (FGD, PLHIV group, Lusaka, April 7, 2011).

The scenario illustrates that dependent agency could have a zero-sum nature: brokers, compliant performers, and/or people who delivered strong extraversion testimonies gained while other individuals lost. As in this example, group leaders who acted as brokers were the winners and often viewed donor projects as a reward for brokering. In the process, they frustrated donors' broader development agenda of ensuring loans so that *many* PLHIV could start a business to earn money for food. When donor interventions are manipulated by local actors who seek to gain the most they can from the situation, the interventions risk becoming irrelevant and ineffective.

The effect of these patterns on donors' relations with local communities could be complicated. On the one hand, donors may refuse to work in communities where dependent agents have used donor projects to benefit themselves. Donor officials may think that community members lack seriousness or accountability (see Patterson 2003), not necessarily recognizing that it is particular dependent agents who have utilized the system to their advantage and not the entire PLHIV group or community. Because donor officials need to report results to their funders, they may shy away from communities with reputations for ineffective projects in which dependent agents have squandered donor resources. One member in the Zambian PLHIV group with the failed loan project explained, "We haven't seen any assistance from donors since the leaders did not pay back" (FGD, PLHIV group, Lusaka, April 7, 2011).

On the other hand, as Chapter 2 indicates, some donors may continue to work with community groups that they know, even if projects in those groups have substandard outcomes. When relationships develop between donors and brokers, and donors feel comfortable with a local group, they may be hesitant to abandon it. After all, they have already invested time in learning about the community and its leaders. Some donors have committed to local groups for the "long haul" and thus, will "walk with them no matter what" (Interviews, FBO partner, Chicago, IL, August 30, 2013;

FBO official, Lusaka, August 15, 2007). Additionally, brokers may be able to explain subpar group performance in ways that donors can accept. For example, several PLHIV group leaders discussed how chicks in their projects died from disease; they did not discuss how (or if) members' negligence may have contributed to this outcome (FGDs, PLHIV groups, Lusaka, March 23, 2011, Kitwe, May 19, 2011; Karonga, August–September 2011; Informal discussion, NGO official, Chingola, May 20, 2011).

The issue of winners and losers goes beyond neighborhood projects, as donor AIDS efforts have created a new class of development entrepreneurs in both countries (Morfit 2011). The "Africa rising" trope includes the argument that Africa is witnessing the growth of a middle class, a demographic category that grew from 200 to 300 million people between 2000 and 2010 (Resnick 2015, 574). While Richard Sklar (1975) defined class in terms of linkages to the African state, more recently scholars have understood class in terms of the individual's role in the service industry, including work with international and national NGOs and FBOs, UN agencies, local businesses, and multinational corporations (Resnick 2015; Barnes et al. 2015). Many such individuals serve as brokers who link the West to African communities and who have benefited from structures of aid dependence. The rise of this group of brokers has occurred at the same time that economic inequality has increased in many African states, including Malawi and Zambia (Mussa and Masanjala 2015; ZIPAR 2013, iv).

Second, dependent agents challenge the neoliberal assumption that all people can be agents in development processes. As illustrated below, we do not deny the capabilities that all individuals bring to their development trajectories. But the aforementioned unequal outcomes illustrate that certain capabilities matter more than others in dependent aid structures. Confidence, English language skills, the willingness to tell one's AIDS story, the willingness to literally or figuratively dress the part, and knowledge about how to stretch the rules on budgets or policies were essential skills. Performances required knowing the script, or the words and actions that donor officials want to hear. Phrases like "All we want is to be empowered"; "If we just had a little capital we could start a small business"; and "We just need skills and then we will stand on our own" must be learned (FGDs, PLHIV groups, Lusaka, March 30, 2011; April 5, 2011; April 23, 2011; Karonga, August–September, 2011). Yet not everyone had the skills, personality, experiences, or information to be an effective dependent agent. Trainings provided one learning environment, but not everyone was included in trainings (see Watkins and Swidler 2013; Smith 2003; Interview, NAPHAM coordinator, Zomba, June 28, 2011). The inequalities that emerge in terms of who gains "dependent agent skills" illustrate that development projects sometimes may reconfigure existing power structures at all levels of society (see Swidler and Watkins 2009, 1183; Bird-David 1990, 189–196, 1983, 57–86). For example, over time younger, educated individuals with English proficiency have edged out older women for caregiving positions, even though older women had provided much of the AIDS care during the initial years of the epidemic (Iliffe 2006). Younger, educated individuals have been more likely to be chosen for trainings, where they learn performances of compliance and extraversion motifs, skills which then increase the likelihood they will be chosen for additional NGO positions (Interviews, NGO workers, Lusaka, May 5, 2011; May 10, 2011; FBO officials, Lusaka, August 9, 2007; August 15, 2007; Participant observations, PLHIV groups, Zomba and Karonga, June–September 2011). Their language skills and training enable them to serve as brokers who translate donors' biomedical, technocratic approach to caregiving to local PLHIV (Cataldo et al. 2008; Kalofonos 2014; Patterson 2016; see also Dixon and McGregor 2011).

Third, dependent agency counters neoliberalism's emphasis on sustainability (Scherz 2014). The very existence of dependent agents and their success in getting benefits shows a lack of sustainability, since these outcomes come directly because of their relationship with the donor audience. Agency is rooted in a relationship in which each party recognizes the power of the other (see Mann 1994, 100). Dependent agents perform *for someone*; they tell their story *to someone*; they connive around *someone else's* rules. The inequalities embedded in the aid system necessitate local agency, but they also allow local people to benefit. Rather than fostering a system in which their exit is possible because the projects they support will continue without them, donors reward the individuals who benefit from existing development structures. Even if the system rewards new players who have donor-preferred skills (like younger, educated caregivers), the larger aid system that sustains a relationship between donors and dependent agents remains (Krause 2014).

A goal of sustainable AIDS programs has been to incorporate PLHIV into the response. Because of their unique ability to explain how HIV and AIDS affect physical health and social relationships (Paxton 2002), HIV prevention programs have relied on PLHIV to educate community members about HIV transmission and testing (Interviews, NGO official,

Lusaka, May 5, 2011; NAPHAM coordinator, Zomba, June 28, 2011). Additionally, many PLHIV become caregivers because of a sense of duty toward other PLHIV, their religious faith, and/or hope for material and social rewards (Maes 2014). Yet local inequalities that emerge from dependent agency may undermine such participation. Donors must be aware of the needs and views of all potential participants, not just the dependent agents who may be better equipped to share their ideas or demonstrate their commitment. And donors must understand how dependent agents may benefit from externally funded programs while other community members do not. These lessons stretch beyond AIDS programs to other health and development initiatives that demand long-term commitments from community members.

DEPENDENT AGENCY AND LOCAL DEMOCRACY

Even though Malawi and Zambia have become more democratic since the early 1990s, as Gabrielle Lynch and Gordon Crawford (2011) write about Africa more generally, they continue to experience centralization of power, endemic corruption, ethnic-based voting, weak civil society organizations, limits on civil liberties, uneven development, and the "perverse" impact of donor–recipient relationships on democratization. Lynch and Crawford (2011, 295) highlight how donor involvement cultivates "a narrow set of elite NGOs who lack democratic credentials themselves, yet have the capacity to act as proxies for donors in influencing the policies of elected governments in ways that remain consistent with donors' own policy choices, that is economic liberalization and private sector development." Democratization can contribute to the reproduction of neopatrimonial relationships that enhance political power and threaten democratic consolidation (Lindberg 2003). Furthermore, donors can become embroiled within the failures of democratization, and donor officials can become apologists for the lack of democratic progress (Brown 2011). At the local level, the exclusionary nature of donor–recipient relationships may erode trust and solidarity. Here we drill down to the impact of dependent agency on local democracy with respect to citizenship responsibilities and democratic deepening.

Citizenship Responsibilities

In both countries, citizens seem hesitant to hold government accountable, to view government officials as political equals, and to express their political views. While they participate in electoral politics, citizens have not embraced the full extent of their citizenship role (Bratton and Logan 2013, 198). For example, a sizeable minority of Zambians think a good citizen should avoid criticizing government (35 %), should agree with the majority opinion in the community (41 %), and should ask elected officials for help in paying for personal expenses like funeral costs (77 %). For 41 % of Zambians and 32 % of Malawians, efficient provision of government services is more important than government accountability to citizens (Afrobarometer 2014, 17–22, 2013a, 16–23). How might dependent agency relate to these views on citizenship?

Democratization efforts have tended to emphasize a liberal view of citizenship, or one which envisions a vertical relationship between the state and autonomous individuals. The state ensures the rights of individuals who are defined to be citizens by legal requirements, and individuals participate in politics to hold the state accountable for protecting those rights (Bratton and Logan 2013; Marshall 1964, 78; Dorman et al. 2007). In newly democratic states, citizens often learn about their rights through donor-directed, top-down processes that emphasize global norms like the "right to development" and the "right to health." Governmentality, or the structures through which the state controls bodies, relies on such empowered, politically conscious citizens (UN 1986; OHCHR and WHO 2008; Roalkvam 2014, 5–7).

Dependent agency may contradict these assumptions about liberal citizenship in several ways. First, dependent agents are not autonomous actors, trained through donor-driven, top-down processes to govern themselves in apolitical processes. Instead, they are enmeshed in webs of interdependence that lead them to engage in strategies of extraversion, performances of compliance, and resistance below the line to gain benefits. They may politicize the very top-down, empowerment processes such as citizenship trainings that donors support. In the process, the "development of citizens" becomes less about fostering liberal citizens and more about empowering communal citizens whose identity is tied to gaining benefits for a select group (Turner 1993, 12–15; Patterson 1999). Second, liberal citizenship assumes that participation to hold government accountable will benefit all citizens, since it ensures that government protects citizens' rights. Yet even though dependent agents may use "rights language" in extraversion and performances of compliance, their focus on rights is not necessarily to promote the rights of all. Instead, as Chapter 3 indicated, rights talk becomes part of extraversion jargon that seeks benefits for a few.

Third, liberal citizenship focuses on the state, but as Bettina Von Lieres (2014, 49) asserts, in marginalized communities citizenship is not experienced in relation to the state but instead "through highly localised processes of horizontal identification and mobilisation." Dependent agents in Zambia and Malawi rarely made demands on state officials, because they realized that the state did not provide the majority of health care funding and that the state was largely absent in the daily workings of their lives (van de Walle 2001). For example, of the 57 Zambian PLHIV and caregiving groups we studied, only seven advocated to state officials. Recognizing the state's lack of material resources, only three of the seven groups requested material benefits such as the provision of ARVs at a local clinic and the purchase of a CD4 machine. In contrast, members in all Zambian groups used some type of agentic strategies with external partners (PLHIV groups, Lusaka, Kitwe, Ndola, Mumbwa, Livingstone, Kabwe, March–June 2011; June 2014). If dependent agents can gain benefits from donors, why should they monitor state actions between elections, contact state officials, or mobilize to demand state services? Citizens' attention to donors instead of the state requires us to rethink notions of liberal citizenship that undergird democratization projects in Africa.

Dependent Agency and Democratic Deepening

In addition to problematizing liberal citizenship, dependent agents may have complicated and contradictory effects on democratic deepening. On one hand, through their under-the-radar actions that have the potential to influence donor processes, dependent agents engage in the politics of accountability. They mobilize individually or collectively for more responsive programs or material resources, illustrating a form of political participation (Scott 1990). Susan Thomson (2014) views agentic moves against the authoritarian Rwandan government as a form of citizenship, because they are rooted in notions of rights and responsibilities. Similarly, one PLHIV in Zambia commented that by voicing their needs to donors at trainings through strategies of extraversion and performances of compliance, local people are able to help donors "better understand our situations and to design good projects" (Interview, PLHIV, Ndola, June 9, 2014).

On the other hand, the actions of dependent agents may not promote mass attitudes like trust, participation, accountability, transparency, and political equality that are essential to sustain democracy (Putnam 1994;

Ingelhart and Welzel 2005). Because we examined the values of trust and solidarity in the context of economic development, we focus here on transparency, accountability, and political equality though we recognize how these values intertwine to shape both socioeconomic and political development. The following case study from Malawi demonstrates how dependent agency can embody and perpetuate undemocratic practices.

One of the authors and a district NGO representative chatted informally in a small market in rural Zomba in 2011 after their visit with a CBO. When the author had first formally interviewed the NGO representative at his office, he had elaborated about the NGO's work to empower communities of PLHIV. As she became more acquainted with the representative, however, the author learned that the NGO was experiencing funding challenges and that, because of Malawi's fuel crisis, the representative had not visited the communities he was supposed to help in months. He had co-opted the project-provided motorbike as his own private vehicle, and despite his official rhetoric, the project was no longer operating. In fact, the author and NGO representative only visited the CBO because the author had bought fuel and insisted on the visit. During the CBO meeting, group members praised the project's benefits, and they did not ask about the NGO's withdrawal of support in the author's presence. Instead the CBO chair took the NGO representative aside to privately raise the issue of funding. In his informal discussion with the author after this meeting, the NGO representative criticized the CBO for complaining about the lost NGO support. At the same time, he defended his decision to ensure his personal gains from the project by retaining his relatively comfortable salary and use of the project laptop and motorbike. He sought to maximize NGO opportunities, because he knew that the project would soon end and he feared losing the relatively comfortable lifestyle he had come to enjoy. He had friends who had worked for other NGOs who had suffered such a fate (Participant observation, CBO meeting, Namasalima, Zomba, July 7, 2011).

The themes of lack of accountability, limited transparency, and hierarchical, elitist attitudes embedded in this case study were evident in our observations, FGDs, and interviews in both countries (Participant observations, FGDs, interviews, PLHIV, caregivers, and donor officials, Lusaka, Ndola, Kitwe, Mumbwa, Livingstone, Zomba, and Karonga, March–September 2011). From this case study and our broader fieldwork, we draw multiple lessons. First, local brokers like the NGO official may lack accountability to the very people they are supposed to represent. As a linkage between the NGO and the local community, the Malawian NGO official was not accountable to the CBO. This lack of accountability derived from the fact that he controlled information and local people's access to donor resources. Brokers "are supposed to represent *the* local populations, express its [sic] 'needs' to the structures in charge of aid ... In fact, far from being passive operators of the logic[s] of dependence, development brokers are *the* key actors in the irresistible hunt for projects carried out in and around African villages" (Bierschenk et al. 2002, 4; emphasis in original). It is through the broker that the Malawian CBO could (or could not) receive funding. Because power was centralized in the broker, it was difficult to hold that person accountable. Local people want connections to donors, and they perceive that brokers with appropriate language and cultural skills are essential to facilitate such linkages. Thus if brokers act in arbitrary or capricious ways, local people may not question them (Patterson 2003). In the case study, the group does not ask publicly why their funding has ended but the NGO representative still has his job. While they may not have wanted to embarrass the representative, they also did not want to burn a broker-facilitated bridge to current or future donors.

Second, dependent agency is fueled by a lack of transparency among all parties in the development web. As the NGO representative performed for the author, he disguised the true nature of his community work. The CBO engaged in similar performances, making it difficult to know its actual activities. The NGO representative did not tell the CBO about his personal use of NGO resources, and the CBO chair did not raise the issue of NGO funding publicly so that all CBO members would know about the money situation. The NGO itself did not communicate its financial difficulties to the villagers. In this context of rumors, suppositions, and omitted information, dependent agents have the power to shape the narrative and control who has the information to hold leaders accountable.

Third, hierarchies that emerge among donors, brokers, and local people may facilitate elitist attitudes which, in turn, undermine trust and political equality (Putnam 1994). As he complained about the CBO's funding demands, the NGO official questioned the villagers' right to actively participate in the development processes that affect them. And by not publicly holding the NGO official accountable, the villagers bought into these hierarchical relationships in which local people depend on those above them to act as patrons who ensure their survival. These patterns resemble neopatrimonial rule in which "big men" act through personal networks to make arbitrary decisions that benefit the people or groups they favor (Médard 1982; Bach and Gazibo 2012; Beresford 2015).

Yet, it is crucial to recognize that brokers like the Malawian NGO worker are situated precariously on the "fault lines and connection points within complex systems and relationships" (Lewis and Mosse 2006, 12). On the one hand, they have obligations that require them to gain benefits for kith and kin. On the other hand, unequal power relations with donors make them vulnerable to arbitrary decisions and an unplanned loss of a job and/or resources. Their position is also murky because donors reward individuals based not on objective criteria like economic need but instead on performances of compliance and extra-version stories. Charismatic brokers who can use neoliberal jargon on human rights, entrepreneurship, and empowerment have a greater chance to benefit than others who do not play the game (Nguyen 2010; Mosse and Lewis 2005). In our observations, articulate and charismatic brokers contrasted with dozens of PLHIV who were shy around strangers, spoke little English, and could not clearly articulate an AIDS story (Interviews and FGDs, PLHIV, and PLHIV groups, Kabwe, Lusaka, Kitwe, Livingstone, Lilongwe, Zomba, and Karonga, February–September 2011). Yet these donor-connected brokers seemed no more or less needy than the other PLHIV. The lack of transparency about the criteria that donors used to reward local people led some groups to claim that donors had favorites (FGDs and PLHIV groups, Lusaka, March 9–10, 2011; Karonga, August–September 2011).

Donor and recipient states have committed to strengthening participatory practices that involve a broad range of development partners (OECD 2008, 8), and they have agreed that "openness, trust, and mutual respect and learning lie at the core of effectiveness in support of development goals" for "intended beneficiaries" (OECD 2011, 3). Because these statements have been supported by state actors, they may ignore the "behind the scenes" ways that dependent agents influence transparency, participation, and accountability in development processes. Donor and recipient states must recognize how they ultimately rely on local people who are enmeshed in webs of uneven power hierarchies and social obligations. Thus even as donors promote aid efficiency by working through brokers who "speak donors' language," they may undermine local accountability and participatory decision-making and reinforce notions of favoritism based on intangible characteristics. Such practices make consolidation of democracy more problematic.

In summary, the presence of potential donor benefits in the lives of PLHIV in Malawi and Zambia means that citizenship is framed not in terms of actions aimed at the state in order to ensure rights, but rather as actions that target donors. In the process, the state may claim credit for donors' activities, and citizens may even give it credit, as Audrey Sacks (2012) discovered in the case of ARV access in several African states. This pattern of upward accountability creates professional projects and delivers results, but it "detracts from grassroots empowerment in that it binds implementing agencies operating in dynamic environments to goals and values of actors higher up in the aid network" (Dixon and Andrew 2011, 1370). The outcome of donor–local interactions, therefore, may be the creation of hybrid forms of accountability that complicate the role of citizens in governance. The creation of "webs of multiple accountabilities that bind the different parties involved" contribute to "competing claims of (il)legitimacy" (Dixon and Andrew 2011, 1370). Since they do not target the state, dependent agents may undermine the long-term development of responsible citizens who call for accountable and transparent governance. And as donor programs reward some local agents over others based on unclear criteria, they perpetuate the favoritism and lack of transparency that undermines long-term democratic consolidation.

Lessons on Conceptual Complexity: Dependent Agency and International Politics

Despite long-established work within African studies, which asserts Africa's agency within powerful structures of globalization (Bayart 2000; Cooper 2001, 190), the continent tends to remain peripheral in the study of international relations (Death 2015). Africa's marginalization is evident in several ways. First, Africa has often been ignored because of its limited economic and military power, being portrayed as a pawn in neoliberal development strategies or global conflict. Second, the field's use of a structural lens has obscured the agentic behavior of African actors who are embedded within those structures (Clapham 1996). Third, Western conceptual frameworks have tended to be applied to African cases based on an assumption "that international regimes, institutions, laws, norms, and values originate in 'the West' and spread out thence to the periphery" (Death 2015, 1–2; see also Harman and Brown 2013; Chabal and Daloz 1999, 142). As Simon Rushton (2005, 450) asserts, in the field of global health, this tendency translates into [policy] models and understandings of what represents an appropriate healthcare system, and how such services should be financed and delivered. Thus recipient states are "taught" not only how health policy should be made (for example, through a centralised Ministry of Health with overall responsibility for national health policy) but also, and perhaps more insidiously, what the resultant policies should be.

As a result, policies often are inappropriately designed and implemented in the African context.

Even when Africa is seriously considered in the politics of global health (see Brown et al. 2009; Cornelissen et al. 2012), the analysis has been limited to relatively powerful states, particularly South Africa. For example, Jeremy Youde (2005) argues that the counterepistemic community of the South African government translated history and identity into policy outcomes that challenged the established discourse on international AIDS control, while Garrett Brown (2014, 878) showed how global health norms were significantly "glocalised" by South African actors. Our analysis moves beyond these trends by taking African agency seriously, approaching grassroots activities through the lens of local actors, and showing the existence of agency among impoverished people in poor states that are dependent on donor funding.

Our actor-oriented approach also contributes to theories of African agency through the concept of *dependent agency*. We seek to move discussions of local agency beyond normative judgments to challenge scholars and practitioners to appreciate the complexity of the "arts of resistance." Because of dependent agency's seemingly "hidden" and apolitical nature, our analysis requires a degree of interpretation that leads to a set of tentative conclusions (Chabal 2014; Scott 1990). First, agency and dependency are not, despite appearances, mutually exclusive. These phenomena run along a continuum, since agents operate within existing power structures. Work within African studies has long established that despite the structural constraints of dependency that emanate from colonialism, unequal globalization processes, and the unequal distribution of global power, African actors may engage in diverse forms of agentic behavior (Lonsdale 2000). They practice a "constant strategic alertness" in their search for opportunities, which may only be possible because of the very inequalities embedded in the international aid system (Sivaramakrishnan 2005, 350; see also Bayart 2000, 218).

Malawi and Zambia illustrate how agency is possible in extreme cases of poverty and aid dependency, the least likely places one might expect to find agentic behavior. In both countries, life is precarious and there are narrow margins for survival, especially with the intersecting economic, food, and HIV crises. And yet, despite people's lived situations of insecurity, many are surviving and some are flourishing, including PLHIV who have faced economic despondency, near-death experiences, social stigma, and family ostracism. Unable to change these structures of economic and social dependence, local people learn to navigate these obstacles in order to survive and, in some cases, even achieve upward social mobility.

Second, dependent agency is fluid. Even though Zambians and Malawians are situated in very tight corners of poverty and dependency, these corners are not static. Chapter 2 examined how the AIDS enterprise expanded and then retracted its programs and funding as donors reacted to corruption scandals in Malawi and Zambia and as they moved from an emergency response to one focused on sustainability. Chapter 3 then illustrated how actors developed diverse agentic behaviors as the conditions of dependency changed over time. For example, local agents used extraversion strategies to complain about their exclusion from donor projects, or they stressed their Christian compassion when donor funding declined or food parcels ended. They learned to play the game over time, as they adopted the structures (e.g., meetings, reports, and rules), technologies (e.g., testimony giving), and jargon (e.g., discourses on positive living and rights) that donors valued.

Dependent agents' various identities were also fluid constructs in these dynamic conditions. Particular identities could bring opportunities at crucial moments. As we illustrated, PLHIV identity brought benefits, but sometimes it alone was insufficient to gain donors' attention. As Chapter 3 showed, being a woman, living in a particular geographic location, or being an MSM sometimes could open doors for resources to subgroups of PLHIV. Dependent agents responded to these fluctuating preferences. They joined church caregiving groups, women's PLHIV groups, or pretended to be MSM at different points in time. Yet, because donors and dependent agents function through an unequal relationship, when local players prioritized particular identities, they could shape donor processes. For example, when large numbers of people claimed to be PLHIV, donors started to ask questions about potential recipients' identities (Interview, donor official, Lusaka, March 31, 2011).

Third, dependent agency is highly political. Here we mean "political" in its most basic form: who benefits and who loses in decision-making over resource allocation, representation, and the acceptance of hegemonic values (Lasswell 1936). Even though dependent agents target donors (not the state) and their strategies do not overturn power structures, their small activities do affect who wins and who loses in environments where the smallest victory may bring food for hungry family members, status, or employment. Dependent agents are acutely aware of power and inequalities, "exercising tactical forms of compliance that give the appearance of obedience... in ways that translate into collective political consciousness" (Thomson 2014, 106). Their awareness of the ability to manipulate, maneuver, and subtly critique donor structures and policies illustrates consciousness, and their engagement in political strategies such as framing issues, negotiating with players, and translating demands between donors and locals is intensely political.

In addition, their actions help underscore the complexity of power, or the currency which drives particular outcomes. Power is never absolute, but rather a relationship rooted in the consent of the ruled: "power is enabling, it provides common people with the chance to create opportunities"; it is not static or "a privilege that some have and others do not" (Bleiker 2000, 61). While donors use resources as a tool of power in order to shape local people's actions, their power ultimately rests on the legitimacy that dominated people give to donors and their programs. Dependent agents play a crucial role in supporting (in the case of performances of compliance and extraversion) or undermining (in the case of resistance below the line) that legitimacy. The strategies of dependent agents teach us not only about dissent but more crucially about the structures and values of the existing order. We learn, for example, how the existing order creates openings for such actions and the reasons why the leaders of the existing order may or may not respond to those actions (Dreyfus and Rabinow 1993, 210–211). Donors only have power over local people's actions to the extent that dependent agents agree to that power and can benefit in tangible and intangible ways from it. Recognizing the political nature and power dynamics of dependent agency helps to elucidate local patterns of inclusion and exclusion. These individual- and community-level lessons must become more integrated into the study of global health politics, a field which has tended to focus on institutional structures (Kamradt-Scott 2015), coordination of various actors in governance (Fidler 2007), technical and management solutions (Lee et al. 2002), and health as a security concern (McInnes 2006; Elbe 2006, 2009, 2010; Price-Smith 2009; McInnes and Rushton 2010;

Nunes 2013). The study of local agency contributes nuanced explanations for why institutional policies do not always work, actors cannot be easily coordinated, technical solutions fail, and state security may do little to foster human security (Davies 2009).

Even though dependent agency is political, it is not necessarily progressive. There may be a "nefarious exercise of agency" that leads to material inequalities, lack of transparency, poor accountability, project failures, and stagnated development trajectories (Chabal 2014, xviii). Such outcomes occur because dependent agents have incentives to maintain the status quo, since it is the current system of aid dependence that brings resources in the absence of an African state that often lacks the capacity and accountability to provide for the basic health and development of citizens (Englebert 2009). Dependent agents do not challenge the aid architecture; rather they hope to tweak it along the margins.

Finally, dependent agency informs the capabilities approach to development (Sen 1985; Sen and Nussbaum 1993), an approach that moves beyond merely focusing on quantitative achievement (e.g., GDP growth or number of people on ARVs) to questioning the promotion of basic decency and justice. It focuses on choice and freedom and respects people's power for self-definition as they "subvert others' expectations" about their actions (Thomson 2014, 111). Capabilities are a type of substantial freedom, "not just abilities residing inside a person but also the freedoms or opportunities created by a combination of personal abilities and the political, social and economic environment" (Nussbaum 2011, 20). Our analysis of dependent agents illustrates the complex, tangled knot of personal characteristics, contextual situations, and societal structures which comprise capabilities. By showing how dependent agents utilize such capabilities to create their own development trajectories, we recognize that even the most marginalized people desire some level of dignity in their struggle for survival (Thomson 2014, 115). We met dozens of such individuals—the compliant district NGO worker who uses the language of rights and gets invited to international AIDS conferences; the AIDS caregiver who leaves a training a little early (after getting her per diem), claiming she is needed at home; the HIV-negative person who pretends to be HIV positive despite the AIDS stigma because he needs food parcels for his family. While these dependent agents do not change global power structures, they are able to act, react, speak, and remain silent in ways that makes their lives just a little bit better in the tight corners of poverty and aid dependence.

NOTE

1. CD4 refers to a specific protein found on the surface of white blood cells and necessary for immune defense. The CD4 count is widely used to measure the level of immune suppression in an HIV-positive person.

BIBLIOGRAPHY

African Development Bank. 2014. *African Economic Outlook (AEO)*. http://www.africaneconomicoutlook.org/en. Accessed January 17, 2016.

African Development Bank. 2015. *Zambia*. http://www.africaneconomicoutlook.org/fileadmin/uploads/aeo/2015/CN_data/CN_Long_EN/Zambia_GB_2015.pdf. Accessed January 17, 2016.

AfDB. *See* African Development Bank.

Afrobarometer. 2012. *Summary of Results Round 5 Malawi*. http://afrobarometer.org/sites/default/files/publications/Summary%20of%20results/mlw_r5_sor.pdf. Accessed November 13, 2014.

Afrobarometer. 2013a. *Zambia Round 5 Summary of Results*. http://www.afrobarometer.org/publications/zambia-round-5-summary-results-2013. Accessed November 13, 2014.

Afrobarometer. 2013b. *Trust and Corruption in Zambia: Results from the Afrobarometer Round 5*. http://www.afrobarometer.org/files/documents/media_br iefing/zam_r5_presentation3.pdf. Accessed November 15, 2014.

Afrobarometer. 2014. *Summary of Results: Afrobarometer Round 6. Survey in Zambia 2014*. http://afrobarometer.org/sites/default/files/publications/Summary%20of%20results/zam_r6_sor_en.pdf. Accessed October 3, 2014.

Aggleton, P., S. A. Bell, and A. Kelly-Hanku. 2014. "Mobile Men with Money": HIV Prevention and the Erasure of Difference. *Global Public Health* 9(3): 257–270.

Andersen, Hans Christian. 1837. *The Emperor's New Clothes*. Trans. Jean Hersholt. http://www.andersen.sdu.dk/vaerk/hersholt/TheEmperorsNewClothes_e.html. Accessed April 15, 2016.

Anderson, Emma-Louise. 2012. Infectious Women: Gendered Bodies and HIV in Malawi. *International Feminist Journal of Politics* 14(2): 267–287.

© The Author(s) 2017   113
E.-L. Anderson, A.S. Patterson, *Dependent Agency in the Global Health Regime*, DOI 10.1057/978-1-137-58148-8

Anderson, Emma-Louise. 2015. *Gender, Risk and HIV: Navigating Structural Violence*. Basingstoke: Palgrave MacMillan.

Anderson, Emma-Louise, and Alexander Beresford. 2016. Infectious Injustice: The Political Foundations of the Ebola Crisis in Sierra Leone. *Third Word Quarterly* 37(3): 468–486.

Ayittey, George. 1999. *Africa in Chaos*. New York: Palgrave Macmillan.

Bach, Daniel, and Mamoudou Gazibo, eds. 2012. *Neopatrimonialism in Africa and Beyond*. New York: Routledge.

Barnes, Amy, Garrett Brown, and Sophie Harman. 2015. *Global Politics of Health Reform in Africa: Performance, Participation and Policy*. Basingstoke: Palgrave Macmillan.

Barnett, Michael, and Martha Finnemore. 2004. *Rules for the World: International Organizations in Global Politics*. Ithaca: Cornell University Press.

Barnett, Tony, and Gwyn Prins. 2006. HIV/AIDS and Security: Fact, Fiction and Evidence—A Report to UNAIDS. *International Affairs* 82(2): 359–368.

Bartlett, David. 2000. Civil Society and Democracy: A Zambian Case Study. *Journal of Southern African Studies* 26(3): 429–446.

Bayart, Jean-François. 2000. Africa and the World: A History of Extraversion. *African Affairs* 99(395): 217–267.

Baylies, Carolyn, and Janet Bujra, eds. 2000. *AIDS, Sexuality and Gender in Africa: Collective Strategies and Struggles in Tanzania and Zambia*. London: Routledge.

Beckmann, Nadine, and Janet Bujra. 2010. The "Politics of the Queue": The Politicization of People Living with HIV/AIDS in Tanzania. *Development and Change* 41(6): 1041–1064.

Benton, Adia. 2015. *HIV Exceptionalism: Development through Disease in Sierra Leone*. Minneapolis: University of Minnesota Press.

Beresford, Alexander. 2015. Power, Patronage and Gatekeeper Politics in South Africa. *African Affairs* 114(455): 226–248.

Bierschenk, Thomas, Jean-Pierre Chauveau, and Jean-Pierre Olivier de Sardan. 2002. *Local Development Brokers in Africa: The Rise of a New Social Category*. Working Paper 13. Department of Anthropology and African Studies. Mainz: Johannes Gutenberg University. http://www.ifeas.uni-mainz.de/Dateien/Local.pdf. Accessed March 27, 2016.

Bird-David, Nurit. 1983. Wage-Gathering: Socio-Economic Change and the Case of the Naiken of South India. In *Rural South Asia: Linkages, Changes and Development*, ed. Peter Robb, 57–89. London: Curzon Press.

Bird-David, Nurit. 1990. The Giving Environment: Another Perspective on the Economic System of Gatherer-Hunters. *Current Anthropology* 1(2): 189–196.

Bleiker, Roland. 2000. *Popular Dissent, Human Agency and Global Politics*. New York: Cambridge University Press.

Boesten, Jelke. 2011. Navigating the AIDS Industry: Being Positive and Poor in Tanzania. *Development and Change* 42(3): 781–803.

Branch, Adam, and Zachariah Mampilly. 2015. *Africa Uprising: Popular Protest and Political Change*. London: Zed Books.

Bratton, Michael. 1992. Zambia Starts Over. *Journal of Democracy* 3(2): 81–94.

Bratton, Michael. 1999. Political Participation in a New Democracy: Institutional Considerations from Zambia. *Comparative Political Studies* 32(5): 549–588.

Bratton, Michael, and Carolyn Logan. 2013. Voters but Not Yet Citizens: The Weak Demand for Vertical Accountability. In *Voting and Democratic Citizenship in Africa*, ed. Michael Bratton, 197–215. Boulder: Lynne Rienner Press.

Brown, Garrett W. 2014. Norm Diffusion and Health System Strengthening. *Review of International Studies* 40(5): 877–896.

Brown, Stephen. 2011. "Well, What Can You Expect?": Donor Officials' Apologetics for Hybrid Regimes in Africa. *Democratization* 18(2): 512–534.

Brown, William. 2012. A Question of Agency: Africa in International Politics. *Third World Quarterly* 33(10): 1889–1898.

Brown, William, and Sophie Harman. 2013. *African Agency in International Politics*. London: Routledge.

Bunker, Stephen. 1987. *Peasants Against the State: The Politics of Market Control in Bugisu, Uganda, 1900–1983*. Chicago: University of Chicago Press.

Burchardt, Marian. 2013. Faith-Based Humanitarianism: Organizational Change and Everyday Meanings in South Africa. *Sociology of Religion* 74(1): 30–55.

Bush, George W. 2003. State of the Union Address. January 28. http://www.washingtonpost.com/wp-srv/onpolitics/transcripts/bushtext_012803.html. Accessed April 3, 2009.

Cataldo, F., K. Kielmann, M. Musheke, and Virginia Bond. 2008. New Challenges for Home-based Care Providers in the Context of ART Rollout in Zambia. Unpublished paper presented at the XVII International AIDS Society Conference, Mexico City, August 3–8.

Central Intelligence Agency. 2015a. *World Factbook: Malawi*. https://www.cia.gov/library/publications/the-world-factbook/geos/mi.html. Accessed October 1, 2015.

Central Intelligence Agency. 2015b. *World Factbook: Zambia*. https://www.cia.gov/library/publications/the-world-factbook/geos/za.html. Accessed October 1, 2015.

Chabal, Patrick. 2014. Forward. In *Arts of Resistance in the 21st Century*, ed. Ebenezer Obadare and Wendy Willems, xii–xviii. London: James Currey.

Chabal, Patrick, and Jean-Pascal Daloz. 1999. *Africa Works: Disorder as Political Instrument*. Bloomington: Indiana University Press.

Chabal, Patrick, Ulf Engle, and Leo de Haan, eds. 2007. *African Alternatives*. Leiden: Brill.

Chambers, Robert. 1997. *Whose Reality Counts? Putting the First Last*. London: ITDG Publishing.

Cheyeka, Austin. 2009. Towards a History of the Charismatic Churches in Post-Colonial Zambia. In *One Zambia, Many Histories*, ed. Jan-Bart Gewald, Marja Hinfelaar, and Giacomo Macola, 144–163. Leiden: Brill.

Chimwaza, A. F., and S. C. Watkins. 2004. Giving Care to People with Symptoms of AIDS in Rural Sub-Saharan Africa. *AIDS Care* 16(7): 795–807.

Chinsinga, Blessings. 2003. Lack of Alternative Leadership in Democratic Malawi: Some Reflections Ahead of the 2004 General Elections. *Nordic Journal of African Studies* 12(1): 1–22.

Chinsinga, Blessings. 2007. District Assemblies in a Fix: The Perils of Self-Seeking Tendencies in Decentralization Policy Reforms in Malawi. *Africa Development* XXXII 1: 89–111.

CIA. *See* Central Intelligence Agency.

Clapham, Christopher. 1985. *Third World Politics: An Introduction*. London: Croom Helm.

Clapham, Christopher. 1996. *Africa and the International System: The Politics of State Survival*. Cambridge: Cambridge University Press.

Coleman, James. 1988. Social Capital and the Creation of Human Capital. *American Journal of Sociology* 94(Supplement): S95–S120.

Cooper, Frederick. 2001. What Is the Concept of Globalization Good For? An African Historian's Perspective. *African Affairs* 100(399): 189–213.

Cornelissen, Scarlett, Fantu Cheru, and Timothy M. Shaw. 2012. Introduction. In *Africa and International Relations in the Twenty-First Century*, ed. Scarlett Cornelissen, Fantu Cheru, and Timothy Shaw, 1–20. Basingstoke: Palgrave Macmillan.

Davies, Sarah. 2009. *Global Politics of Health*. Malden: Polity Press.

Davies, Sarah, Adam Kamradt-Scott, and Simon Rushton. 2015. *Disease Diplomacy: International Norms and Global Health Security*. Baltimore: The Johns Hopkins University Press.

De Bruijn, Marjam, Rijk van Dijk, and Jan-Bart Gewald. 2007. Social and Historical Trajectories of Agency in Africa. In *African Alternatives*, ed. Patrick Chabal, Ulf Engle, and Leo de Haan, 9–20. Leiden: Brill.

De Bruijn, Marjam E., and Han J. W. M. Van Dijk. 1999. Insecurity and Pastoral Development in the Sahel. *Development and Change* 30(1): 115–139.

De Smedt, Johan. 2009. "No Raila, No Peace!" Big Man Politics and Election Violence at the Kibera Grassroots. *African Affairs* 108(433): 581–598.

Death, Carl. 2015. Introduction: Africa's International Relations. *African Affairs*. Online Only Exclusive Article. https://www.oxfordjournals.org/our_journals/afrafj/death_africa_international_relations.pdf. Accessed April 20, 2016.

Department for International Development Malawi. 2012a. Support to the Extended National HIV and AIDS Action Framework—Business Case. March. https://www.iati.dfid.gov.uk/iati_documents/3717550. docx. Accessed January 17, 2016.

Department of International Development Malawi. 2012b. *Operational Plan 2011–2015*. May. https://www.gov.uk/government/uploads/system/uploads/attach ment_data/file/67387/malawi-2011.pdf. Accessed January 17, 2016.

DfID Malawi. *See* Department of International Development Malawi.

DiMaggio, Paul J., and Woody W. Powell. 1983. The Iron Cage Revisited: Institutional Isomorphism and Collective Rationality in Organizational Fields. *American Sociological Review* 48: 147–160.

Dionne, Kim. 2012. Local Demand for a Global Intervention: Policy Priorities in the Time of AIDS. *World Development* 40(12): 2468–2477.

Dionne, Kim Yi, Patrick Gerland, and Susan Watkins. 2013. AIDS Exceptionalism: Another Constituency Heard From. *AIDS Behavior* 17(3): 825–831.

Dixon, Rowan, and Andrew McGregor. 2011. Grassroots Development and Upwards Accountabilities: Tensions in the Reconstruction of Aceh's Fishing Industry. *Development and Change* 42(6): 1349–1377.

Dorman, Sara, Daniel Hammett, and Paul Nugent. 2007. *Making Nations, Creating Strangers: State and Citizenship in Africa*. Leiden: Brill.

Dreyfus, Hubert L., and Paul Rabinow. 1993. *Michel Foucault: Beyond Structuralism and Hermeneutics*. 2nd ed. Chicago: University of Chicago Press.

Dunn, Kevin, and Timothy Shaw. 2001. *Africa's Challenge to International Relations Theory*. New York: Palgrave Press.

Economist. 2013. A Hopeful Continent. Special Report: Emerging Africa. *The Economist*, March 2.

Edwards, Michael, and David Hulme. 1996. *Beyond the Magic Bullet: NGO Performance and Accountability in the Post-Cold War World*. West Hartford: Kumarian Press.

Elbe, Stefan. 2006. Should HIV/AIDS be Securitized? The Ethical Dilemmas of Linking HIV/AIDS and Security. *International Studies Quarterly* 50(1): 119–144.

Elbe, Stefan. 2009. *Virus Alert: Security, Governmentality, and the AIDS Pandemic*. New York: Columbia University Press.

Elbe, Stefan. 2010. *Security and Global Health*. Malden: Polity Press.

Ellis, Stephen. 2011. *Season of Rains: Africa in the World*. Chicago: University of Chicago Press.

Ellis, Stephen, and Ineke van Kessel. 2009. *Movers and Shakers: Social Movements in Africa*. Leiden: Brill.

England, Roger. 2007. Are We Spending Too Much on AIDS? *BMJ* 334: 344.

Englebert, Pierre. 2009. *Unity, Sovereignty, Sorrow*. Boulder: Lynne Rienner Publishers.

Englebert, Pierre, and Kevin Dunn. 2013. *Inside African Politics.* Boulder: Lynne Rienner Publishers.

Englund, Harri. 2006. *Prisoners of Freedom: Human Rights and the African Poor.* Berkeley: University of California Press.

Epstein, Helen. 2007. *Invisible Cure: Why We Are Losing the Fight Against AIDS in Africa.* New York: Picador.

Evans, Peter. 1979. *Dependency and Development: The Alliance of Multinational, State and Local Capital.* Princeton: Princeton University Press.

Ferguson, James. 1994. *The Anti-Politics Machine: Development, Depoliticization and Bureaucratic Power in Lesotho.* Minneapolis: University of Minnesota Press.

Ferguson, James. 1999. *Expectations of Modernity: Myths and Meanings of Urban Life on the Zambian Copperbelt.* Los Angeles: University of California Press.

Ferguson, James. 2010. The Uses of Neoliberalism. *Antipode* 41(supplement S1): 166–184.

Ferguson, James. 2013. Declarations of Dependence: Labour, Personhood and Welfare in Southern Africa. *Journal of Royal Anthropological Institute* 19(2): 223–242.

Fidler, David. 2007. Reflections on the Revolution in Health and Foreign Policy. *Bulletin of the World Health Organization* 85(3): 243–244.

Finnemore, Martha. 2009. Legitimacy, Hypocrisy, and the Social Structure of Unipolarity. *World Politics* 61(1): 58–85.

Finnemore, Martha, and Kathryn Sikkink. 1998. International Norm Dynamics and Political Change. *International Organization* 52(4): 887–917.

Fox, Ashley. 2014. AIDS Policy Responsiveness in Africa: Evidence from Opinion Surveys. *Global Public Health* 9(1–2): 224–248.

Freedom House. 2015a. Malawi. https://freedomhouse.org/report/freedom-world/2015/malawi#.VeCyf_lViko. Accessed September 18, 2015.

Freedom House 2015b. Zambia. https://freedomhouse.org/report/freedom-world/2015/zambia#.VeCyU_lViko. Accessed September 18, 2015.

Freston, Paul. 2004. *Evangelicals in Politics in Asia, Africa and Latin America.* New York: Cambridge University Press.

Frueh, Jamie. 2013. Global Messages and Local Spaces: Creativity and Ownership in the Prevention of HIV. Paper Presented at the International Studies Association Conference, Toronto, March 26–29.

Fukuyama, Francis. 1995. *Trust: The Social Virtues and the Creation of Prosperity.* New York: Free Press.

Garmaise, David. 2011. CHAZ to Replace ZNAN as PR for HIV Grants in Zambia; ZNAN No Longer Solvent. *AIDSpan* 116, October 27. http://www.aidspan.org/gfo_article/chaz-replace-znan-pr-hiv-grants-zambia-znan-no-longer-solvent. Accessed November 15, 2015.

Giddens, A. 1984. *The Constitution of Society: Outline of the Theory of Structuration*. Cambridge: Policy Press.

Global Fund. 2010. The Office of the Inspector General Progress Report for March-October 2010 and 2011 Audit Plan and Budget. 22nd Board Meeting, Sofia, December 13–15. http://www.theglobalfund.org/documents/board/22/BM22_09OIG_Report_en/. Accessed September 27, 2016.

Global Fund. 2013. *Zambia Expands Access to Treatment for HIV*. http://www.theglobalfund.org/en/mediacenter/newsreleases/2013-10-17_Zambia_Expands_Access_to_Treatment_for_HIV. Accessed November 16, 2015.

Global Fund. 2014. *Update on Results and Impact*. http://www.theglobalfund.org/en/publications. Accessed September 25, 2016.

Global Fund. 2015a. *Malawi: Financial Information*. http://portfolio.theglobalfund.org/en/Country/Index/MWI. Accessed January 17, 2016.

Global Fund. 2015b. *Zambia: Financial Information*. http://portfolio.theglobalfund.org/en/Country/Index/ZMB. Accessed January 17, 2016.

Global Fund. 2015c. *Zambia: Investments to Date*. http://www.theglobalfund.org/en/portfolio/country/?loc=ZMB. Accessed January 17, 2016.

Global Fund. 2015d. *Zambia and Global Fund Sign $234 Million in New Grants*. http://www.theglobalfund.org/en/news/2015-01-9_Zambia_and_Global_Fund_Sign_$234_Million_in_New_Grants. Accessed January 18, 2016.

GoM. *See* Government of Malawi.

Gould, Deborah. 2009. *Moving Politics: Emotion and ACT UP's Fight against AIDS*. Chicago: University of Chicago Press.

Government of Malawi. 2011. Malawi National HIV and AIDS Strategic Plan 2011–2016. Lilongwe. http://www.safaids.net/files/malawi_national_hiv_and_aids_plan_2011-2016.pdf. Accessed May 5, 2015.

Government of Malawi. 2015. *Malawi AIDS Response Progress Report*. Lilongwe. http://www.unaids.org/sites/default/files/country/documents/MWI_narrative_report_2015.pdf. Accessed May 5, 2015.

Grépin, Karen. 2012. HIV Donor Funding Has Both Boosted and Curbed the Delivery of Different Non-HIV Health Services in Sub-Saharan Africa. *Health Affairs* 31(7): 1406–1414.

Gusman, Alessandro. 2009. HIV/AIDS, Pentecostal Churches and the "Joseph Generation" in Uganda. *Africa Today* 56(1): 66–86.

Harbeson, John, Donald Rothchild, and Naomi Chazan. 1994. *Civil Society and the State in Africa*. Boulder: Lynne Rienner Publishers.

Harman, Sophie. 2009. Fighting HIV and AIDS: Reconfiguring the State? *Review of African Political Economy* 36(121): 343–367.

Harman, Sophie, and William Brown. 2013. In from the Margins? The Changing Place of Africa in International Relations. *International Affairs* 89(1): 69–87.

Harvey, David. 2005. *A Brief History of Neoliberalism*. London: Oxford University Press.

Hawkins, D., D. Lake, D. Nielson, and M. Tierney, eds. 2006. *Delegation Under Anarchy in International Organizations.* New York: Cambridge University Press.

Heywood, Mark. 2009. South Africa's Treatment Action Campaign: Combining Law and Social Mobilization to Realize the Right to Health. *Journal of Human Rights Practice* 1(1): 14–36.

Hilhorst, Dorthea. 2003. *The Real World of NGOs: Discourses, Diversity and Development.* London: ZED Press.

Hodgson, Dorothy. 2011. *Being Maasai, Becoming Indigenous: Postcolonial Politics in a Neoliberal World.* Bloomington: Indiana University Press.

Hungbo, Jendele. 2014. "Beasts of No Nation": Resistance and Civic Activism in Fela Anikulapo-Kuti's Music. In *Arts of Resistance in the 21st Century,* ed. Ebenezer Obadare and Wendy Willems, 167–182. London: James Currey.

Hunsmann, Moritz. 2015. Global Health Initiatives in the Long Run: Donor Responsibility, African Agency and the Sustainability of Antiretroviral Treatment in Tanzania. Paper Presented at the International Studies Association Conference, New Orleans, February 18-21.

Hunter, Susan, and John Williamson. 1997. *Children on the Brink.* Washington, DC: USAID.

Huntington, Samuel. 1968. *Political Order in Changing Societies.* New Haven: Yale University Press.

Hyden, Goran. 1980. *Beyond Ujamaa in Tanzania: Underdevelopment and an Uncaptured Peasantry.* Berkeley: University of California Press.

Hyden, Goran. 2006. *African Politics in Comparative Perspective.* New York: Cambridge University Press.

Igoe, Jim. 2006. Becoming Indigenous Peoples: Difference, Inequality and the Globalization of East African Identity Politics. *African Affairs* 105(420): 399–430.

Iliffe, John. 2006. *The African AIDS Epidemic: A History.* James Currey: Oxford.

Ingelhart, Robert, and Carl Welzel. 2005. *Modernization, Cultural Change and Democracy.* Cambridge: Cambridge University Press.

Jackson, Robert, and Carl Rosberg. 1984. Personal Rule: Theory and Practice in Africa. *Comparative Politics* 14(4): 421–442.

Jalali, Rita. 2013. Financing Empowerment? How Foreign Aid to Southern NGOs and Social Movements Undermines Grass-Roots Mobilization. *Sociology Compass* 7(1): 55–73.

Johnson, Krista. 2006. AIDS and the Politics of Rights in South Africa: Contested Terrain. *Human Rights Review* 7(2): 115–129.

Joint United Nations Programme on HIV/AIDS. 2014. *Fact Sheet 2014.* http://www.unaids.org/sites/default/files/en/media/unaids/contentassets/documents/factsheet/2014/20140716_FactSheet_en.pdf. Accessed July 26, 2015.

Joint United Nations Programme on HIV/AIDS. 2015. *Fact Sheet: 2014 Global Statistics.* http://www.unaids.org/sites/default/files/media_asset/20150714_FS_MDG6_Report_en.pdf. Accessed October 3, 2015.

Kaiser Family Foundation. 2015a, January 23. Data Note: Americans' Views on the U. S. Role in Global Health. http://kff.org/global-health-policy/poll-finding/data-note-americans-views-on-the-u-s-role-in-global-health. Accessed September 24, 2015.

Kaiser Family Foundation. 2015b. Financing the Response to AIDS in Low- and Middle-income Countries. http://kff.org/report-section/financing-the-response-to-aids-in-low-and-middle-income-countries-report. Accessed November 3, 2015.

Kaler, Amy, and Susan Watkins. 2010. Asking God about the Dates You Will Die: HIV Testing as a Zone of Uncertainty in Rural Malawi. *Demographic Research* 23(32): 905–932.

Kalofonos, Ippolytos Andreas. 2010. "All I Eat Is ARVs": The Paradox of AIDS Treatment Interventions in Central Mozambique. *Medical Anthropology Quarterly* 24(3): 363–380.

Kalofonos, Ippolytos Andreas. 2014. "All They Do Is Pray": Community Labour and the Narrowing of "Care" during Mozambique's HIV Scale-Up. *Global Public Health* 9(1–2): 7–24.

Kamradt-Scott, Adam. 2015. *Managing Global Health Security: The World Health Organization and Disease Outbreak Control*. New York: Palgrave MacMillan.

Kapstein, Ethan, and Joshua Busby. 2013. *AIDS Drugs for All: Social Movements and Market Transformations*. Cambridge: Cambridge University Press.

Kassim, H., and A. Menon. 2003. The Principal-Agent Approach and the Study of the European Union: Promise Unfulfilled? *Journal of European Public Policy* 10 (1): 121–139.

Kelly, Kevin J., and Karen Birdsall. 2010. The Effects of National and International HIV/AIDS Funding and Governance Mechanisms on the Development of Civil-Society Responses to HIV/AIDS in East and Southern Africa. *AIDS Care* 22(S2): 1580–1587.

Kemp, Julia, Jean Marion Aitken, Sarah LeGrand, and Biziwick Mwale. 2003. Equity in Health Sector Responses to HIV/AIDS in Malawi. Regional Network for Equity in Health in Southern Africa (EQUINET). Discussion Paper Number 5. http://www.equinetafrica.org/bibl/docs/aidsmalawi.pdf. Accessed November 12, 2015.

Kenworthy, Nora J. 2014. Participation, Decentralization and Déjà Vu: Remaking Democracy in Response to AIDS? *Global Public Health* 9(1–2): 25–41.

Kingsley, Pete. 2014. NGOs, Donors and the Patrimonial State—Tactics for Political Engagement in Nigeria. *Critical African Studies* 6(1): 6–21.

Krakauer, Mark, and Jodie Newbery. 2007. Churches' Responses to HIV/AIDS in Two South African Communities. *Journal of the International Association of Physicians in AIDS Care* 6(1): 27–35.

Krause, Monika. 2014. *The Good Project: Humanitarian Relief NGOs and the Fragmentation of Reason*. Chicago: University of Chicago Press.

Lasswell, Harold. 1936. *Politics: Who Gets What, When, How*. New York: Whittlesey House.

Lee, Kelley. 2004. The Pit and the Pendulum. *Development* 47(2): 11–17.

Lee, Kelley, Kent Buse, and Suzanne Fustukain. 2002. *Health Policy in a Globalising World*. New York: Cambridge University Press.

Lewis, David, and David Mosse. 2006. *Brokers and Translators: The Ethnography of Aid and Agencies*. Westport: Kumarian Press.

Lindberg, Staffan I. 2003. It's Our Time to "Chop": Do Elections in Africa Feed Neopatrimonialism Rather than Counter-Act It? *Democratization* 10(2): 121–140.

Long, Norman. 1990. From Paradigm Lost to Paradigm Regained? The Case for an Actor-oriented Sociology of Development. *European Review of Latin American and Caribbean Studies* 49 (December): 3–24.

Lonsdale, John. 2000. Agency in Tight Corners: Narrative and Initiative in African History. *Journal of African Cultural Studies* 13(1): 5–16.

Lynch, Gabrielle. 2012. Becoming Indigenous in the Pursuit of Justice: The African Commission on Human and Peoples' Rights and the Endorois. *African Affairs* 111(442): 24–45.

Lynch, Gabrielle, and Gordon Crawford. 2011. Democratization in Africa 1990–2010: An Assessment. *Democratization* 18(2): 275–310.

Maes, Kenneth. 2014. "Volunteers Are Not Paid Because They Are Priceless": Community Health Worker Capacities and Values in an AIDS Treatment Intervention in Urban Ethiopia. *Medical Anthropology Quarterly* 29(1): 97–111.

Malawi Vulnerability Assessment Committee. 2012. *National Food Security Assessment*. Lilongwe: MVAC.

Mann, Jonathan. 1999. *Health and Human Rights: A Reader*. New York: Taylor & Francis.

Mann, Patricia. 1994. *Micro-Politics: Agency in a Postfeminist Era*. Minneapolis: University of Minnesota Press.

Marshall, Katherine, and Marisa Van Saanen. 2007. *Development and Faith*. Washington, DC: World Bank.

Marshall, Thomas. 1964. *Class, Citizenship and Social Development*. New York: Doubleday.

Matfess, Hilary. 2015. Developmental Authoritarianism in Rwanda and Ethiopia. *African Studies Review* 58(2): 181–204.

McInnes, Colin. 2006. HIV/AIDS and Security. *International Affairs* 82(2): 315–26.

McInnes, Colin, and Simon Rushton. 2010. HIV, AIDS and Security: Where Are We Now? *International Affairs* 86(1): 225–245.

Médard, Jean-François. 1982. The Underdeveloped State in Tropical Africa: Political Clientelism or Neo-Patrimonialism. In *Private Patronage and Public Power*, ed. Christopher Clapham, 162–191. London: Pinter.

Médicins sans Frontières. 2001. Press Conference, June 26. http://www.un.org/press/en/2001/msfpc.doc.htm. Accessed January 18, 2015.

Médicins sans Frontières. 2011, February 13. Malawi: Challenges Ahead in HIV Treatment, http://www.doctorswithoutborders.org/news-stories/voice-field/malawi-challenges-ahead-hiv-treatment. Accessed May 6, 2015.

Morfit, N. Simon. 2011. "AIDS Is Money": How Donor Preferences Reconfigure Local Realities. *World Development* 39(1): 64–76.

Moser, Caroline, O. 1989. Gender Planning in the Third World: Meeting Practical and Strategic Gender Needs. *World Development* 17(11): 1799–1825.

Mosse, David, and David Lewis, eds. 2005. *The Aid Effect: Giving and Governing in International Development*. London: Pluto Press.

MSF. *See* Médicins sans Frontières.

Mussa, Richard, and Windford Henderson Masanjala. 2015. *A Dangerous Divide: The State of Inequality in Malawi*. Report for Oxfam. https://www.oxfam.org/sites/www.oxfam.org/files/file_attachments/rr-inequality-in-malawi-261115-en.pdf. Accessed January 17, 2016.

MVAC. *See* Malawi Vulnerability Assessment Committee.

Mwandawire, Thandika. 2015. Neopatrimonialism and the Political Economy of Economic Performance in Africa: Critical Reflections. *World Politics* 67(3): 563–612.

NAO. *See* National Audit Office.

National Audit Office. 2009, October 30. *Department for International Development: Aid to Malawi*. NAO: London.

National Statistics Office and ICF Macro. 2011. *Malawi Demographic and Health Survey* (MDHS), 2010, Zomba. http://dhsprogram.com/pubs/pdf/FR247/FR247.pdf. Accessed May 5, 2015.

Ndulo, Manenga, Dale Mudenda, Lutangu Ingombe, and Frank Chansa. 2010. *Global Financial Crisis Discussion Series Paper 22: Zambia Phase 2*. Report for Overseas Development Institute. http://www.odi.org/sites/odi.org.uk/files/odi-assets/publications-opinion-files/5798.pdf. Accessed January 19, 2015.

Nepstad, Sharon Erickson. 2011. *Nonviolent Revolutions: Civil Resistance in the Late 20th Century*. New York: Oxford University Press.

Newell, Jonathan. 1995. "A Moment of Truth"? The Church and Political Change in Malawi, 1992. *Journal of Modern African Studies* 33(2): 243–262.

Nguyen, Vinh-Kim. 2010. *The Republic of Therapy*. Durham: Duke University Press.

Nguyen-Krug, Helena, and Hans Hogerzeil. 2006. Human Rights: A Potentially Powerful Force for Essential Medicines. *Bulletin of the World Health Organization* 84(5): 410–411.

NSO. *See* National Statistics Office.

Ntata, Pierson R. 2007. Equity in Access to ARV Drugs in Malawi. *SAHARA J (Journal of Social Aspects of HIV/AIDS Research Alliance)* 4 (1): 564–574.

Nunes, João. 2013. *Security, Emancipation and the Politics of Health: A New Theoretical Perspective.* Abingdon: Routledge.

Nussbaum, Martha. 2011. *Creating Capabilities: The Human Development Approach.* Cambridge, MA: Belknap Press.

OECD. *See* Organisation for Economic Co-operation and Development.

Office of the Inspector General. 2012. *Audit of the Global Fund Grants to the Republic of Malawi.* August. Lilongwe: Global Fund/OIG.

Office of the United Nations High Commission for Human Rights and World Health Organization. 2008. The Right to Health. Fact Sheet 31. http://www.ohchr.org/Documents/Publications/Factsheet31.pdf. Accessed March 15, 2016.

OHCHR. *See* Office of the United Nations High Commission for Human Rights

OIG. *See* Office of the Inspector General.

Olesen, T. 2006. In the Court of Public Opinion: Transnational Problem Construction in HIV/AIDS Medicine Access Campaign, 1998–2001. *International Sociology* 21(1): 5–30.

Onuf, Nicholas. 2003. Parsing Personal Identity: Self, Other, Agent. In *Language, Agency and Politics in a Constructed World*, ed. François Debrix, 26–49. Armonk: M.E. Sharpe.

Organisation for Economic Co-operation and Development. 2008. *The Paris Declaration on Aid Effectiveness and the Accra Agenda for Action.* http://www.oecd.org/dac/effectiveness/34428351.pdf. Accessed March 17, 2016.

Organisation for Economic Co-operation and Development (OECD). 2011. *Busan Partnership for Effective Development Cooperation. Fourth High Level Forum on Aid Effectiveness.* http://www.oecd.org/development/effectiveness/49650173.pdf. Accessed March 17, 2016.

Organisation for Economic Co-operation and Development. 2013. Aid to Developing Countries Rebounds in 2013 to Reach an All-Time High. http://www.oecd.org/newsroom/aid-to-developing-countries-rebounds-in-2013-to-reach-an-all-time-high.htm. Accessed January 18, 2016.

Ottaway, Marina. 1999. *Africa's New Leaders: Democracy or State Reconstruction?* Washington, DC: Carnegie Endowment for International Peace.

Patterson, Amy. 1999. The Dynamic Nature of Citizenship and Participation: Lessons from Three Rural Senegalese Case Studies. *Africa Today* 46(1): 3–27.

Patterson, Amy. 2003. Power Inequalities and the Institutions of Senegalese Development Organizations. *African Studies Review* 46(3): 35–54.

Patterson, Amy. 2006. *The Politics of AIDS in Africa.* Boulder: Lynne Rienner Publishers.

Patterson, Amy. 2011. *The Church and AIDS in Africa: The Politics of Ambiguity.* Boulder: FirstForum Press.

Patterson, Amy. 2013. Pastors as Leaders in Africa's Religious AIDS Mobilisation: Cases from Ghana and Zambia. *Canadian Journal of African Studies* 47(2): 207–226.

Patterson, Amy. 2015. Engaging Therapeutic Citizenship and Clientship: Untangling the Reasons for Therapeutic Pacifism among People Living with HIV in Urban Zambia. *Global Public Health* 10: 1–14.

Patterson, Amy. 2016. Training Professionals, Eroding Relationships: Donors, AIDS Care, and Development in Urban Zambia. *Journal of International Development* 28(6): 827–844.

Paxton, Susan. 2002. The Impact of Utilizing HIV-Positive Speakers in AIDS Education. *AIDS Education and Prevention* 14(4): 282–294.

Pearson, Mark. 2010. *Impact Evaluation of the Sector-Wide Approach.* DfID Human Development Resource Centre. https://www.gov.uk/government/uploads/sys tem/uploads/attachment_data/file/67670/imp-eval-sect-wde-appr-mw. pdf. Accessed December 17, 2016.

Peiffer, Caryn, and Pierre Englebert. 2012. Extraversion, Vulnerability to Donors, and Political Liberalization in Africa. *African Affairs* 111(444): 355–378.

PEPFAR. *See* President's Emergency Plan for AIDS Relief.

Peters, P.E. 1992. Against All Odds: Matriliny, Land and Gender in the Shire Highlands. *Critique of Anthropology* 17(2): 189–210.

Pitcher, Anne, Mary Moran, and Michael Johnston. 2009. Rethinking Patrimonialism and Neopatrimonialism in Africa. *African Studies Review* 52(1): 125–156.

Population Council. 2010. RAPIDS Evaluation Final Report 2005–2009. http://www.popcouncil.org/uploads/pdfs/2010HIV_RAPIDSEval.pdf. Accessed January 8, 2016.

Posner, Daniel. 2004. The Political Salience of Cultural Difference: Why Chewas and Tumbukas Are Allies in Zambia and Adversaries in Malawi. *American Political Science Review* 98(4): 529–545.

President's Emergency Plan for AIDS Relief. 2011. *Partnership to Fight HIV/AIDS in Zambia.* http://www.pepfar.gov/countries/zambia. Accessed November 1, 2015.

President's Emergency Plan for AIDS Relief. 2013. Sustainability Guidance Planning Document: Advancing Country Ownership in PEPFAR III. http://www.pepfar.gov/documents/organization/217767.pdf. Accessed November 7, 2015.

President's Emergency Plan for AIDS Relief. 2014. *Partnering to Achieve Epidemic Control in Malawi.* http://www.pepfar.gov/documents/organiza tion/199568.pdf. Accessed March 7, 2016.

President's Emergency Plan for AIDS Relief. 2015. Ambassador's Welcome. http://zambia.usembassy.gov/pepfar.html. Accessed March 1, 2016.

President's Emergency Plan for AIDS Relief. 2016. Partnering to Achieve Epidemic Control in Malawi. http://www.pepfar.gov/countries/malawi. Accessed March 7, 2016.

Price-Smith, Andrew. 2009. *Contagion and Chaos: Disease, Ecology and National Security in the Era of Globalization*. Cambridge, MA: MIT Press.

Putnam, Robert. 1994. *Making Democracy Work*. Princeton: Princeton University Press.

Putzel, James. 2004. The Global Fight Against AIDS: How Adequate Are the National Commissions? *Journal of International Development* 16(8): 1129–1140.

Ranger, Terence. 1995. *Are We Not Also Men? The Samkange Family and African Politics in Zimbabwe, 1920–1964*. London: James Currey.

Rasmussen, Louise Mubanda. 2013. "To Donors It's a Program, But to Us It's a Ministry": The Effects of Donor Funding on a Community-Based Catholic HIV/AIDS Initiative in Kampala. *Canadian Journal of African Studies* 47(2): 227–247.

Rau, Bill. 2006. The Politics of Civil Society in Confronting HIV/AIDS. *International Affairs* 82(2): 285–295.

Ravelo, Jenny Lei. 2012. In Zambia, A Global Fund Grant for HIV. *Development Newswire*. October 11. https://www.devex.com/news/in-zambia-a-global-fund-grant-for-hiv-response-79420. Accessed January 7, 2016.

Reno, Will. 1998. *Warlord Politics and African States*. Boulder: Lynne Rienner Publishers.

Resnick, Danielle. 2011. In the Shadow of the City: Africa's Urban Poor in Opposition Strongholds. *Journal of Modern African Studies* 49(1): 141–166.

Resnick, Danielle. 2015. The Political Economy of Africa's Emergent Middle Class: Retrospect and Prospects. *Journal of International Development* 27: 573–587.

Reubi, David. 2011. The Promise of Human Rights for Global Health: A Programmed Deception? *Social Science and Medicine* 73: 625–628.

Roalkvam, Sidsel. 2014. Health Governance in India: Citizenship as Situated Practice. *Global Public Health* 9(8): 1–17.

Robins, Steven. 2004. "Long Live Zackie. Long Live!" AIDS Activism, Science and Citizenship after Apartheid. *Journal of Southern African Studies* 30: 651–672.

Root, Robin, and Arnau van Wyngaard. 2011. Free Love: A Case Study of Church-Run Home-Based Caregivers in a High Vulnerability Setting. *Global Public Health* 6(supplement 2): S174-S191.

Rostow, Walt. 1960. *The Stages of Economic Growth: A Non-Communist Manifesto*. New York: Cambridge University Press.

Rushton, Simon. 2005. Health and Peacebuilding: Resuscitating the Failed State in Sierra Leone. *International Relations* 19: 441–456.

Sacks, Audrey. 2012. *Can Donors and Non-State Actors Undermine Citizens' Legitimating Beliefs?* Afrobarometer Working Paper 140. http://afrobarometer. org/publications/can-donors-and-non-state-actors-undermine-citizens%E2%80% 99-legitimating-beliefs. Accessed April 18, 2014.

Scherz, China. 2014. *Having People, Having Heart: Charity, Sustainable Development and Problems of Dependence in Central Uganda*. Chicago: University of Chicago Press.

Schratzberg, Michael. 2001. *Political Legitimacy in Middle Africa: Father, Family, Food*. Bloomington: Indiana University Press.

Scott, James. 1990. *Domination and the Arts of Resistance*. New Haven: Yale University Press.

Seckinelgin, Hakan. 2008. *The International Politics of HIV/AIDS: Global Disease— Local Pain*. London: Routledge.

Seekings, J., and N. Nattrass. 2005. *Class, Race and Inequality in South Africa*. New Haven: Yale University Press.

Sen, Amartya. 1985. *Commodities and Capabilities*. Oxford: Oxford University Press.

Sen, Amartya, and Martha Nussbaum, eds. 1993. *The Quality of Life*. Oxford: Clarendon Press.

Sexuality Information and Education Council of the US. 2008. 2008 PEPFAR Country Profile Update: Zambia. http://www.siecus.org/index.cfm?fuseac tion=page.viewPage&pageID=969&nodeID=1. Accessed October 12, 2015.

Shiffman, Jeremy. 2008. Has Donor Prioritization of HIV/AIDS Displaced Aid for Other Health Issues? *Health Policy and Planning* 23(2): 95–100.

Shiffman, Jeremy, David Berlan, and Tamara Hafner. 2009. Has Aid for AIDS Raised All Health Funding Boats? *JAIDS* 52(Supplement 1): S45–S48.

SIECUS. *See* Sexuality Information and Education Council of the US.

Simutanyi, Neo. 2013. Zambia: Manufactured One-Party Dominance and Its Collapse. In *One-Party Dominance in African Democracies*, ed. Renske Doorenspleet and Lia Nijzink, 119–142. Boulder: Lynne Rienner Publishers.

Siplon, Patricia. 2013. Can Charity and Rights-Based Movements Be Allies in the Fight Against HIV/AIDS? Bridging Mobilisations in the United States and Sub-Saharan Africa. *Canadian Journal of African Studies* 47(2): 187–205.

Siplon, Patricia, and Kristin Novotny. 2007. Overcoming the Contradictions: Women, Autonomy and AIDS in Tanzania. In *The Global Politics of AIDS*, ed. Paul Harris and Patricia Siplon, 87–107. Boulder: Lynne Rienner Publishers.

Sivaramakrishnan, K. 2005. Some Intellectual Genealogies for the Concept of Everyday Resistance. *American Anthropologist* 107(3): 346–355.

Sklar, Richard. 1975. *Corporate Power in an Africa State: The Political Impact of Multinational Mining Companies in Africa.* Berkeley: University of Berkeley Press.

Skovdal, M., C. Campbell, C. Madanhire, Z. Mupambireyi, C. Nyamukapa, and S. Gregson. 2011. Masculinity as a Barrier to Men's Use of HIV Services in Zimbabwe. *Globalization and Health* 7: 1–14.

Smith, Daniel Jordan. 2003. Patronage, Per Diems and the "Workshop Mentality": The Practice of Family Planning Programs in Southeastern Nigeria. *World Development* 31(4): 703–715.

Smith, J. H., and Alan Whiteside. 2010. The History of AIDS Exceptionalism. *Journal of the International AIDS Society* 3: 13–47.

Swidler, Ann, and Susan Cotts Watkins. 2009. "Teach a Man to Fish": The Sustainability Doctrine and Its Social Consequences. *World Development* 37 (7): 1182–1196.

Syed, Javid. 2011. PLHIV Demand for CCM to Take Action on Disbusement [*sic*] of Funds to Civil Society. Blog post, August 2. https://lists.mayfirst.org/pipermail/tbhiv/2011-August/000410.html. Accessed January 17, 2015.

Szeftel, Morris. 2000. "Eat with Us": Managing Corruption and Patronage Under Zambia's Three Republics, 1964–99. *Journal of Contemporary African Studies* 18(2): 207–224.

Taylor, Ian. 2009. *China's New Role in Africa.* Boulder: Lynne Rienner Publishers.

Taylor, Scott. 2006. Divergent Politico-Legal Responses to Past Presidential Corruption in Zambia and Kenya: Catching the "Big Fish" or Letting Him off the Hook? *Third World Quarterly* 27(2): 281–301.

Thomson, Susan. 2014. Accepting Authoritarianism? Everyday Resistance as Political Consciousness in Post-Genocide Rwanda. In *Civic Agency in Africa: Arts of Resistance in the 21st Century,* ed. Ebenezer Obadare and Wendy Williams, 104–124. London: James Currey.

Tocco, Jack Ume. 2010. "Every Disease Has Its Cure": Faith and HIV Therapies in Islamic Northern Nigeria. *African Journal of AIDS Research* 9(4): 383–395.

Turner, Brian. 1993. *Citizenship and Social Theory.* London: SAGE.

UN. *See* United Nations.

UNAIDS. *See* Joint United Nations Programme on HIV/AIDS.

UNDP. *See* United Nations Development Programme.

United Nations. 1986. *Declaration on the Right to Development.* General Assembly Resolution A/RES/41/128. http://www.un.org/documents/ga/res/41/a41r128.htm. Accessed November 21, 2015.

United Nations. 2001. *Declaration of Commitment on HIV/AIDS.* http://www.unaids.org/sites/default/files/sub_landing/files/aidsdeclaration_en_0.pdf. Accessed October 12, 2013.

United Nations Development Programme. 2013a. *Human Development Report: The Rise of the South—Malawi.* http://hdr.undp.org/sites/default/files/ Country-Profiles/MWI.pdf. Accessed October 9, 2015.

United Nations Development Program. 2013b. *Human Development Report: The Rise of the South—Zambia.* http://hdr.undp.org/sites/default/files/ Country-Profiles/ZMB.pdf. Accessed October 9, 2015.

US State Department. 2015. *Map of Foreign Assistance Worldwide.* http://beta. foreignassistance.gov/explore. Accessed October 21, 2015.

van de Walle, Nicolas. 2001. *African Economies and the Politics of Permanent Crisis.* New York: Cambridge University Press.

van der Veen, A. Maurits. 2011. *Ideas, Interests and Foreign Aid.* New York: Cambridge University Press.

Vander Meulen, Rebecca, Amy Patterson, and Marian Burchardt. 2013. HIV/AIDS Activism, Framing and Identity Formation in Mozambique's. *Equipas de Vida. Canadian Journal of African Studies* 47(2): 249–272.

Von Lieres, Bettina. 2014. Citizenship from Below: The Politics of Citizen Action & Resistance in South Africa & Angola. In *Civic Agency in Africa: Arts of Resistance in the 21st Century,* ed. Ebenezer Obadare and Wendy Willems, 49–62. London: James Currey.

Warren, M.E., ed. 1999. *Democracy and Trust.* Cambridge: Cambridge University Press.

Watkins, Susan Cotts, and Ann Swidler. 2013. Working Misunderstandings: Donors, Brokers and Villagers in Africa's AIDS Industry. *Population and Development Review* 38(Supplement): 197–208.

Wendt, Alexander. 1987. The Agent-Structure Problem in International Relations Theory. *International Organization* 41(3): 383–392.

WFP. *See* World Food Programme.

WHO. *See* World Health Organization.

Whyte, Susan, Michael Whyte, Lotte Meinert, and Jenipher Twebaze. 2013. Therapeutic Clientship: Belonging in Uganda's Projectified Landscape of AIDS Care. In *When People Come First: Critical Studies in Global Health,* ed. João Biehl and Adriana Petryna, 140–165. Princeton: Princeton University Press.

Wilkinson, Annie, and Melissa Leach. 2014. Briefing: Ebola—Myths, Realities, and Structural Violence. *African Affairs* 114(454): 136–148.

William, Brown, Sophie Harman, Stephen Hurt, Donna Lee, and Karen Smith. 2009. Editorial: New Directions in International Relations and Africa. *The Round Table* 98(402): 263–267.

Wilson, Nicolas. 2016. Antiretroviral Therapy and Demand for HIV Testing: Evidence from Zambia. *Economics and Human Biology* 21: 221–240.

World Bank. 2014. World Bank Indicators: Net ODA Received. http://data.world bank.org/indicator/DT.ODA.ODAT.XP.ZS. Accessed October 27, 2015.

World Bank. 2015a. Malawi. http://data.worldbank.org/country/ malawi. Accessed November 3, 2015.

World Bank. 2015b. Zambia. http://data.worldbank.org/country/ zambia. Accessed November 3, 2015.

World Food Programme. 2014. *The State of Food Insecurity in the World*. http:// www.fao.org/3/a-i4030e.pdf. Accessed November 17, 2015.

World Food Programme. 2015. Zambia. http://www.wfp.org/countries/zam bia/overview. Accessed November 4, 2015.

World Health Organization, United Nations Children's Fund, and Joint United Nations Programme on HIV/AIDS. 2013. *Global Update on HIV Treatment: Results, Impact and Opportunities*. http://www.unaids.org/sites/default/files/ sub_landing/files/20130630_treatment_report_en_3.pdf. Accessed September 22, 2015.

Wroe, Daniel. 2012. Donors, Dependency and Political Crisis in Malawi. *African Affairs* 11(442): 135–144.

Wrong, Michela. 2010. *It's Our Time to Eat: The Story of a Kenyan Whistleblower*. New York: Harper Perennials.

Youde, Jeremy. 2005. The Development of a Counter-Epistemic Community. *International Relations* 19: 421–439.

Youde, Jeremy. 2008. Is Universal Access to Antiretroviral Drugs an Emerging International Norm? *Journal of International Relations and Development* 11(4): 415–440.

Zambia NAC. *See* Zambia National AIDS Council.

Zambia Institute for Policy Analysis and Research. 2013. The Distribution of Household Income and the Middle Class in Zambia. Working Paper 14, December. http://elibrary.acbfpact.org/acbf/collect/acbf/index/assoc/ HASH0181.dir/doc.pdf. Accessed October 7, 2015.

Zambia National AIDS Council. 2014. *Zambia Country Report: Monitoring the Declaration of Commitment on HIV and AIDS and Universal Access*. http:// www.unaids.org/sites/default/files/country/documents/ZMB_narrative_ report_2014.pdf. Accessed November 4, 2015.

ZIPAR. *See* Zambia Institute for Policy Analysis and Research.

LIST OF FIELDWORK DATA

INTERVIEWS

Malawi

FBO official, Lilongwe, July 12, 2007
Action Aid official, Lilongwe, July 17, 2007
FBO official, Limbe, July 20, 2007
WFP official, Lilongwe, July 23, 2007
FBO official, Lilongwe, July 24, 2007
CIDA official, Lilongwe, July 26, 2007
CIDA technical advisor, Lilongwe, July 26, 2007
CIDA specialist, Lilongwe, July 27, 2007
DfID official, Lilongwe, July 27, 2007
World Bank official, Lilongwe, July 27, 2007
NAPHAM official, Lilongwe, June 16, 2011
NGO AIDS coordinator, Zomba, June 28, 2011
NAPHAM coordinator, Zomba, June 28, 2011
PLHIV, Zomba City, July 17, 2011
NGO representative, Zomba, July 22, 2011
Donor official, Lilongwe, June 26, 2014
MoF civil servant, Lilongwe, June 26, 2014
MoH civil servant, Lilongwe, June 28, 2014
NGO official, Lilongwe, July 4, 2014
MoF civil servant, Lilongwe, July 27, 2014

© The Author(s) 2017
E.-L. Anderson, A.S. Patterson, *Dependent Agency in the Global Health Regime*, DOI 10.1057/978-1-137-58148-8

Donor HIV expert, Lilongwe, July 26, 2014
Donor technical advisor, Lilongwe, July 27, 2014
PLHIV, Makunganya, Zomba, July 29, 2011

Zambia

FBO official, Lusaka, August 9, 2007
Donor official, Lusaka, August 12, 2007
Bilateral donor, Lusaka, August 13, 2007
Zambia NAC official, Lusaka, August 14, 2007
DfID official, Lusaka, August 15, 2007
FBO official, Lusaka, August 15, 2007
CHAZ official, Lusaka, August 16, 2007
NZP+ official, Lusaka, August 17, 2007
ZNAN official, Lusaka, August 20, 2007
NGO official, Lusaka, April 15, 2009
CHAZ official, Lusaka, April 16, 2009
Donor official, Lusaka, February 23, 2011
PLHIV, Lusaka, February 24, 2011
Church AIDS coordinator, Lusaka, February 25, 2011
PLHIV, Lusaka, March 1, 2011
AIDS clinic counsellor, Lusaka, March 2, 2011
PLHIV, Lusaka, March 2, 2011
PLHIV, Lusaka, March 8, 2011
NGO official, Lusaka, March 17, 2011
NZP+ leader, Lusaka, March 21, 2011
PLHIV, Lusaka, March 22, 2011
PLHIV, Lusaka, March 30, 2011
FBO official, Lusaka, March 31, 2011
FBO official, Lusaka, April 1, 2011
FBO official, Lusaka, April 8, 2011
NZP+ leader, Mumbwa, April 15, 2011
NZP+ leader, Kabwe, April 18, 2011
PLHIV, Lusaka, May 4, 2011
NGO worker, Lusaka, May 5, 2011
PLHIV, Lusaka, May 9, 2011
NGO worker, Lusaka, May 10, 2011
NZP+ official, Lusaka, May 10, 2011
PLHIV, Lusaka, May 10, 2011

NGO official, Kitwe, May 20, 2011
FBO official, Ndola, May 20, 2011
NZP+ leader, Ndola, May 22, 2011
PLHIV, Mpika, July 4, 2011
FBO trainee, Ndola, June 6, 2014
PLHIV, Ndola, June 9, 2014

Other

World Vision official, Washington, DC, April 14, 2005
FBO partner, Minneapolis, MN, August 21, 2013
FBO partner, Chicago, IL, August 30, 2013
AIDS policy expert, Washington, DC, April 15, 2005

FOCUS GROUP DISCUSSIONS

Malawi

PLHIV group, Chiseu, Zomba, July 25, 2011
PLHIV group, Nambande, Zomba July 26, 2011
PLHIV group, Zomba City, July 27, 2011
PLHIV group, Nanchenga, Zomba, July 28, 2011
PLHIV group, Makunganya, Zomba, July 29, 2011
PLHIV group, Nkolokosa, Zomba, July 30, 2011
PLHIV group, Namadi Trading Centre, Zomba, August 1, 2011
PLHIV group, Near Nsondole, Zomba, August 2, 2011
PLHIV group, Nsondole, Zomba, August 3, 2011
PLHIV group, St Agnes Catholic Church, Zomba, August 4, 2011
PLHIV group, TA Kutamanje, Zomba, August 5, 2011
PLHIV group, Chinawali Anglican Church, Zomba, August 6, 2011
PLHIV group, Karonga Boma, Karonga, August 20, 2011
PLHIV group, Kasowa, Karonga, August 22, 2011
PLHIV group, Puse, Karonga, August 23, 2011
PLHIV group, Mwenitete, Karonga, August 24, 2011
PLHIV group, Nbande, Karonga, August 25, 2011
PLHIV group, Lupembe, Karonga, August 26, 2011
PLHIV group, Nyungwe, Karonga, August 27, 2011
PLHIV group, Uliwa, Karonga, August 30, 2011
PLHIV group, Ngara, Karonga, August 31, 2011

PLHIV group, Chilumba Galizon, Karonga, September 1, 2011
PLHIV group, Fuliwira, Karonga, September 2, 2011
PLHIV group, Chilumba, Karonga, September 3, 2011

Zambia

PLHIV groups, Lusaka, February 25, March 2, March 8–10, March 22–24, March 30, April 1, April 5, April 7, April 14, April 23, May 9, 2011
Caregiver group, Lusaka, April 7, 2011
PLHIV group, Kabwe, April 18, 2011
Caregiver group, Kitwe, May 19, 2011
PLHIV group, Kitwe, May 19, 2011
Caregiver group, Ndola, May 21, 2011
PLHIV groups, Ndola, May 22–23, 2011
PLHIV group, Livingstone, June 27, 2011
PLHIV group, Ndola, June 11, 2014

PARTICIPANT OBSERVATIONS

Malawi

MANET+ trainings, Mponela, June 2011
NAPHAM trainings, Zomba City, June 27–29, 2011
PLHIV groups, Zomba and Karonga, June-September 2011
MANASO trainings, Zomba City, July 2011
PLHIV group, Nsondole, Zomba, July 6, 2011
CBO meeting, Namasalima, Zomba, July 7, 2011
District Interfaith Alliance trainings, Karonga Boma, Karonga, August 2011
NAPHAM executive meeting, Karonga Boma, August 19, 2011
NGO training group, Kasowa, Karonga, August 22, 2011
PLHIV group, Karonga, August 22, 2011
Public forums with HIV stakeholders, Lilongwe, June-July 2014;

Zambia

Church service, Lusaka, August 5, 2007
AIDS clinic, Lusaka, March 9–13, 2011
PLHIV group, Lusaka, March 30, 2011

PLHIV groups, Lusaka, Kitwe, Ndola, Mumbwa, Livingstone, Kabwe, March-June 2011; June 2014
PLHIV–author encounter, Lusaka, May 10, 2011
PLHIV group, Ndola, June 9, 2014

INDEX

A
Access to ART
  in Malawi and Zambia, 25, 40
  norms, 19–20
Activists
  donors, 37, 56
  fund rejection, 54
  fund scandal, 67
  human rights, 19–20, 43, 67–68
  and norms of access, 20–21
  and performances of
    compliance, 56–57
  Western policymakers, 12
Actor-oriented approach, 7, 107
Africa rising, 13, 98
Agency
African agency, 4, 5–9, 89, 107–111
  dependent Agency, 2–4, 8–9, 21,
    51, 87–111
  human initiative, 7, 16
  in tight corners, 2, 51, 88, 107–108
AIDS enterprise, 17–21, 34–35, 88
AIDS exceptionalism, see HIV
  exceptionalism
AIDS funding

donor, 17–18
  ramping up in mid 2000s, 35–44
  slowing down after 2009, 45–49
Anti-politics machine, 14, 91
Authenticity
  authentic African role, 15
  authentic groups, 41–42, 44, 75, 80

B
Bayart, François Jean, 13, 14, 55, 88
Becoming HIV positive peoples, 14, 70
Becoming indigenous peoples, 13
Brokers
  and democratic
    deepening, 103–105
  and the AIDS enterprise, 15–16, 44
  aspirations of, 16
  and complaints about
    exclusion, 77–78
  and donor relations, 97–98
  and extraversion, 77–78
  and performances of
    compliance, 59–61, 64
  and resistance below the line, 83

© The Author(s) 2017
E.-L. Anderson, A.S. Patterson, *Dependent Agency in the Global
Health Regime*, DOI 10.1057/978-1-137-58148-8

role of, 15–16, 44, 51, 55, 60–61,
  64, 69, 70, 83, 85, 98
  as winners, 97–99

C
Capabilities approach, 110–111
Case studies, 21–26
  economic situations, 22–24
  ethnic groups, 22
  HIV and AIDS situations, 24–26
  political experiences, 24
Christian compassion, 12, 68, 92, 108
Churches
  and AIDS care, 16, 37, 84
  CHAZ see Churches Health
    Association of Zambia (CHAZ)
Churches Health Association of
  Zambia (CHAZ), 37
  as brokers, 44, 78
  leadership role, 40
  and PLHIV, 26, 78, 96
  in Zambia, 20, 30, 37–38, 41, 67, 95
Clients
  HIV positive people, 14, 17, 38, 40,
    70, 95
  of patrons, 5, 60, 90, 104
Corruption, 33–35, 45–47, 92–93
Country Coordinating
  Mechanism, 17, 37

D
Democracy
  and accountability, 89, 101,
    102–105, 106
  and autonomy, 101
  and citizenship, 100–102
  civil society role in re-establishing
    democracy, 37
  democratic consolidation, 100, 106
  democratic deepening, 100, 102–106

and donors, 102
and hierarchical attitudes, 103,
  104–105
transition to, 36
and transparency, 89, 102, 104
Dependency
  as a joint venture, 14
  as a mode of action, 14
  perceptions of African
    dependency, 13
  theory, 6
Dependent agency
  conditions for, 9–10, 33–52, 88
  definition of, 2–3, 88
  and democratic
    deepening, 102–106
  and development, 89–100
  donor responses to, 51, 90–93,
    97–98
  implications of, 89
  and international politics, 106–111
  and local democracy, 100–106
  as political, 108–110
Dependent agents
  strategies of, 10–17, 53–85, 88
  objectives of, 7, 30, 54, 88
Development
  and theories of agency, 5–7
  and dependent agency, 89–100
  neoliberal, 25, 96, 106
  socioeconomic, 7
Donor
  competition between, 9–10, 41
  donor's eyes on the ground, 92
  responses to dependent agency, 51,
    92–93, 97–98

E
Emergency response, 18, 34–35, 108
Empowerment, 12, 13, 49–51, 56, 66,
  67, 73–74, 89, 101, 105, 106

Exclusion, 19, 75–78, 80, 85, 88, 91, 100, 108–109
Exceptionalism, *see* HIV exceptionalism
Extraversion, 13–14, 69–80, 88–89, 91–92
 of the authentic PLHIV support group, 75
 and brokers, 77–78
 as a "conservative strategy,", 14
 definition of, 13, 55
 of exclusion, 75–78
 donor reactions to, 89, 91–92
 of the diseased body, 70
 of gender, 71–73
 of the healthy, empowered PLHIV, 73–74
 of the marginalized PLHIV, 70–71
 as a "mode of action,", 14, 80
 and socioeconomic advancement, 96
 strategies, 13–14, 69–80, 88
 by training, 79–80
 for training, 78–79

F
Financial crisis, 17–18, 45
Food distribution, 42–43, 50, 51, 68, 83

G
Global Fund for AIDS, Tuberculosis and Malaria
 and corruption, 35, 36
 in Malawi, 18, 25, 34, 35, 36
 in Zambia, 18, 25, 33, 34

H
Hidden transcripts, 9, 16, 81, 90
HIV exceptionalism, 18, 75
Hypocrisy, charges of, 12, 67–69

L
Legitimacy
 and accountability, 106
 of brokers, 15
 of donors, 11–12, 21, 67–68, 89, 92, 93, 109
 of groups, 75, 80
Living positively, 11, 43, 57–58

M
Malawi
 case study, 21–26
Malawi Network of People Living with HIV/AIDS (MANET+), 28, 73, 79–80

N
National AIDS Commission (Malawi), 25, 35, 39
National AIDS Council (Zambia), 25, 38
National Association for People Living with HIV and AIDS in Malawi (NAPHAM), 26–29, 48, 50, 57, 59, 61–64, 65, 67, 71, 76, 77–78, 79, 83
Neoliberalism, 96, 99
Neopatrimonialism, 5–6
Network of Zambian People Living with HIV/AIDS (NZP+), 26–28, 59, 63, 64, 65, 75, 77

P

Participatory action research, 12
Performances of compliance, 10–13,
  29–30, 55–69, 88, 89–91
  and activists, 56–57
  and adopting jargon, 11, 55–59
  and adopting donor-
    approved structures, 59
  and brokers, 59–61, 64
  donor responses to, 89–91
  and echoing the official
    story, 10–11, 55–61
  and "free" terminology, 58–59
  and holding more powerful actors to
    account, 11–13
  learning and normalizing
    performances, 61–64
  and "positive living,", 57–58
  perfecting performances, 64–66
  performers' faces grow to fit the
    masks, 11, 29–30
  refusing to learn the ropes, 66
  and socioeconomic
    advancement, 96
  strategies of, 10–13, 55–69, 88
  and trainings, 12–13, 61–64
Positive living
  donors' jargon, 57
  and extraversion, 74
  performance of, 11, 57–58
  and training, 62
  PLHIV testimonies, 74
Power
  African agency, 4, 5–6
  definition of, 109
  dependent agency, 109–110
  donors, 109
  global relations, 3, 89
  local democracy, 100
  subverting power structures, 87, 110
Principal-agent theory, 7
Projectified environment, 41, 75

R

Research design, 26–30
Resistance below the line, 14–15,
  81–84, 88, 92–93
  and brokers, 83
  donor reactions to, 89, 92–93
  by redefining the issue, 15, 83–84
  by stretching the rules, 82–83
  using euphemisms, 81
  using foot dragging, 14–15, 81–82
  and socioeconomic
    advancement, 96
  strategies of, 14–15, 81–84

S

Scott, James, 8–9, 11, 14, 29, 55, 84, 88
Sector-wide approach (SWAp), 39, 47
Solidarity
  dependent agency, 89, 94–96
  PLHIV, 30
  undermining trust and, 94–96
Structure-agency
  debate about, 6
  linkage between, 8
Support groups for PLHIV, 21,
  26–29, 41
Sustainability
  and dependent agency, 99
  doctrine, 12, 49
  and empowerment, 12, 49–51
  pass-on projects, 50
  training, 50

T

Training sessions
  learning and normalizing
    performances, 61–64
  practices that "make everyone
    happy,", 11, 61
Trust
  as condition for democracy, 89, 94

as condition for development, 89, 94
and dependent agency, 89, 94–96,
  100, 104
within PLHIV support groups, 78,
  95–96

U
US President's Emergency Plan for
  AIDS Relief (PEPFAR), 1, 22,
  35–38, 40

V
Vertical programs, 18

Z
Zambia
  case study, 21–26
Zambian National AIDS
  Network (ZNAN), 37, 40,
  44–46, 75, 78